www.bma.org.uk/library

Competency-Based Critical Care

WITHDRAWN
FROM LIBRARY

KT-838-215

WITHDRAWN
FROM LIBRARY

BRITISH MEDICAL ASSOCIATION

0948693

Series Editors

John Knighton, MBBS, MRCP, FRCA
Consultant
Intensive Care Medicine & Anaesthesia
Portsmouth Hospitals NHS Trust
Portsmouth
UK

Paul Sadler, MBChB, FRCA
Consultant
Critical Care Medicine & Anaesthesia
Queen Alexandra Hospital
Portsmouth
UK

Founding Editor

John S.P. Lumley
Emeritus Professor of Vascular Surgery
University of London
London
UK

and

Honorary Consultant Surgeon
Great Ormond Street Hospital for Children NHS Trust (GOSH)
London
UK

Other titles in this series

Renal Failure and Replacement Therapies
edited by *Sara Blakeley*

A. McLuckie

Respiratory Disease and its Management

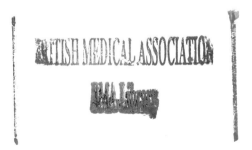
BRITISH MEDICAL ASSOCIATION
BMA Library

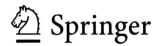
Springer

Angela McLuckie, FRCA, FJFICM
Department of Intensive Care
Guy's and St Thomas' NHS Foundation Trust
London
UK

ISSN: 1864-9998
ISBN: 978-1-84882-094-4   e-ISBN: 978-1-84882-095-1
DOI 10.1007/978-1-84882-095-1
Springer Dordrecht Heidelberg London New York

British Library Cataloguing in Publication Data
A catalogue record for this book is available from the British Library

Library of Congress Control Number: 2009929351

© Springer-Verlag London Limited 2009
Apart from any fair dealing for the purposes of research or private study, or criticism or review,
as permitted under the Copyright, Designs and Patents Act 1988, this publication may only be
reproduced, stored or transmitted, in any form or by any means, with the prior permission in
writing of the publishers, or in the case of reprographic reproduction in accordance with the
terms of licenses issued by the Copyright Licensing Agency. Enquiries concerning reproduction
outside those terms should be sent to the publishers.
The use of registered names, trademarks, etc., in this publication does not imply, even in the
absence of a specific statement, that such names are exempt from the relevant laws and
regulations and therefore free for general use.
Product liability: The publisher can give no guarantee for information about drug dosage and
application thereof contained in this book. In every individual case the respective user must
check its accuracy by consulting other pharmaceutical literature.

Printed on acid-free paper

Springer is part of Springer Science+Business Media (www.springer.com)

Contents

Contributors

Geoffrey J Bellingan, LRCP, MBBS
Centre for Respiratory Research
University College London
London
UK

Andy Bodenham, MBBS, FRCA
Leeds General Infirmary
Leeds
UK

Aimee Brame, MRCP
Department of Critical Care Medicine
Guy's and St Thomas' Hospital
London
UK

Ulrike Buehner, MD, FCARCSI
St James's University Hospital
Leeds
UK

Terry Fox, BSc (Hons) Applied Biology
Department of Critical Care
Guy's and St Thomas' Hospital
London
UK

Michael Gillies, MBChB, FRCA, DICM
Department of Critical Care
Guy's and St Thomas NHS Foundation Trust
London
UK

David Goldhill, MA, MBBS, FRCA, MD, EDIC
Royal National Orthopaedic Hospital
Stanmore, Middlesex
UK

Gerard Gould, FRCA
Department of Anaesthesia
Guy's and St Thomas' Hospital
London
UK

Mark JD Griffiths, MBBS
Adult Intensive Care Unit
Royal Brompton Hospital
London
UK

Nicholas Hart, BSc, MRCP, PhD
Lane Fox Respiratory Unit
Department of Critical Care
Guy's and St Thomas' NHS
Foundation Trust
London
UK

Paul Hayden, MRCP, FRCA, DICM
Department of Anaesthesia
and Critical Care
Medway NHS Foundation Trust
Gillingham, Kent
UK

David CJ Howell, PhD
Centre for Respiratory Research
University College London
London
UK

Andrew Jones, MRCP
Department of Critical Care Medicine
Guy's and St Thomas' Hospital
London
UK

Chris J Langrish, FRCA, MRCP, DICM, EDIC
Guy's and St Thomas' NHS Foundation Trust
London
UK

Richard Leach MD, FRCP
Department of Critical Care
St Thomas' Hospital
London
UK

Philip S Marino, MBBS, BSc (Hons), MRCP (UK)
Respiratory and Critical Care Medicine
Kingston Hospital NHS Trust
Kingston, Surrey
UK

Catherine McKenzie, MRPharmS, PhD
Critical Care and Perioperative Medicine
St Thomas' Hospital
London
UK

George Ntoumenopoulos, BSc BAppSc (Physio), PhD, Grad Dip Clin Epidemiol
Guy's and St Thomas' NHS Foundation Trust
London
UK

John ES Park, MA, MRCP
Adult Intensive Care Unit
Royal Brompton Hospital
London
UK

Adrian Pearce, FRCA
Department of Anaesthesia
Guy's and St Thomas' Hospital
London
UK

Tony Pickworth, MA, BM, BCh, FRCA, FCRP
Department of Anaesthesia
The Great Western Hospital
Swindon
UK

Mansoor Sange MD, DNB, FRCA
Guy's and St Thomas' NHS Foundation Trust
London
UK

David F Treacher FRCP
Department of Intensive Care
Guy's and St Thomas' NHS Foundation Trust
London
UK

Gavin Whelan, MRPharmS, Dip Clin Pharm
St Thomas' Hospital
London
UK

Adrian J Williams, MBBS, FRCP
Lane-Fox Respiratory Unit and Sleep Disorders Centre
St Thomas' Hospital
London
UK

1

Acute Lung Injury and Acute Respiratory Distress Syndrome (ALI/ARDS)

David C.J. Howell and Geoffrey J. Bellingan

Abstract Acute Lung Injury/Acute Respiratory Distress Syndrome (ALI/ARDS) is one of the most devastating conditions that critically ill patients develop. Major advances in understanding the pathogenesis of ALI/ARDS have been made since its initial description in the 1960s. However, the mortality rate for the condition remains high and, to date, there remains no pharmacological therapy that has had an unequivocal benefit in clinical trials.

The aim of this chapter is to discuss current theories on the pathogenesis, diagnosis and various therapeutic strategies available for ALI/ARDS. In addition, it elaborates on all the major contentious issues that exist in this condition.

Introduction

Although there have been huge advances in the overall management of patients with ALI/ARDS since it was first described, many controversial aspects concerning the pathogenesis, diagnosis, therapeutic options and supportive measures for this condition still exist (Table 1.1). ARDS was first described by Ashbaugh in a *Lancet* publication in 1967. However, it is clear from the literature that the condition existed prior to this time (for an excellent recent review, see [1]). There has been some confusion over the years as to what the 'A' in ARDS stands for. Ashbaugh initially referred to it as 'acute' but then modified his description to

'adult', probably to distinguish it from the infant respiratory distress syndrome (IRDS). However, when the American and European Consensus Conference produced the standardised definition of ALI/ARDS [2], which is still used, 'acute' again became the favoured term.

The incidence, or at least diagnosis, of ALI and ARDS appears to be increasing and some reports quote as many as 200,000 cases per year of ARDS in the USA [3, 4]. However, some unpublished key opinions from leaders in the field dispute this as they feel that the incidence of ALI/ARDS is falling. Whatever the true incidence, there is no doubt that mortality of the condition is improving. Historically, mortality rates were around 50–70% but a figure of 30–40% is now more widely quoted (reviewed in [5]). However, this may yet be an overestimate, as the majority of recently published randomised controlled trials (RCTs) quote a 28-day mortality of around 25–30%. It is generally believed that the decrease in mortality over time is due to the improved level of support patients now receive in the intensive care unit (ICU) rather than a specific therapeutic intervention per se. Furthermore, death is not usually related to pulmonary failure, but is rather either a result of the underlying condition that manifested as ALI/ARDS in the first instance or late sepsis.

The aetiology of ALI/ARDS is quite diverse and the disorders associated with clinical development can broadly be divided into those which cause

TABLE 1.1. Current controversies in ALI/ARDS

Controversy	Issue
Pathogenesis	How do the three classical phases of ALI/ARDS interplay?
Diagnosis	Are the diagnostic criteria accurate?
Therapy: Ventilatory strategies	
Tidal volume	How much?
PEEP	High or low?
Recruitment manouevres	Friend or foe?
Prone positioning	Does it have a role?
Modality of ventilation	Does it make any difference?
Complications of ventilation	Are we doing more harm than good?
Therapy: Pharmacological agents	
Steroids	Early, late or not at all?
Surfactant	Tomorrow's saviour?
Nitric oxide	Yesterday's hero?
Support	
Fluid resuscitation	Wet or dry?
Blood transfusion	What effect in ALI/ARDS?
Nutrition	Do calories change prognosis?
Radiology	Chest x-ray or CT?
Surgical lung biopsy	Is it an aid to diagnosis?
Survival post ALI/ARDS	What happens when patients with ALI/ARDS are successfully discharged from ICU?

TABLE 1.2. Aetiology of ALI/ARDS

Direct lung injury	Indirect lung injury
Bronchopneumonia	Sepsis
Gastric aspiration	Multiple trauma with shock
Pulmonary contusion	Drug overdose
Fat emboli	Acute pancreatitis
Inhalational injury	Transfusion-associated acute lung injury (TRALI)
Near-drowning	
Reperfusion injury	Cardiopulmonary bypass

direct lung injury, e.g. bronchopneumonia, or indirect lung injury, e.g. severe trauma (Table 1.2). Interestingly, ALI/ARDS does not consistently develop in patients receiving similar insults. A number of environmental factors such as age, sex, smoking history and pre-existing lung disease are thought to play a role in this observation. However, studies have also shown that polymorphisms in genes, such as the angiotensin-converting enzyme (ACE) gene, produce genotypes that confer protection from the development of ALI/ARDS [9]. It is also thought that certain genotypes may determine the response of the lung to the injurious

effects of mechanical ventilation, which has given rise to the recently coined term, 'ventilogenomics'. Further studies assessing the functional role of candidate genes in ALI/ARDS are awaited with interest and may have a direct influence on the design of clinical trials and therapeutic strategies in the future.

Pathology and Pathogenesis

The pathology and pathogenesis of ALI/ARDS have been discussed in detail in a number of reviews (please see [5, 7]) and will not be elaborated upon in this chapter. Briefly, it is thought that there are three phases: exudative/inflammatory, proliferative and fibrotic (Figure 1.1).

The exudative phase is characterised histologically by diffuse alveolar damage (DAD) as the microvascular endothelial and alveolar epithelium, which form the alveolar–capillary barrier, become disrupted. Following injury, the endothelial barrier becomes extremely permeable leading to highly proteinaceous, haemorrhagic pulmonary oedema fluid flooding into the alveoli, which also leads to fibrinous hyaline membrane formation. Epithelial integrity is also breached, as damage to Type I and II pneumocytes occurs. This leads to exacerbation of alveolar oedema as permeability of the epithelium increases and its resorptive function ceases. In addition, as Type II cells are also injured, surfactant production is reduced. Widespread neutrophilic infiltration is a major feature in this phase.

During the proliferative phase, further capillary network damage is evident and intimal proliferation occurs in small blood vessels. Necrosis of Type I pneumocytes leads to exposure of the epithelial basement membrane and Type II cells proliferate in an attempt to repair the damage. Fibrinous exudates become organised and are replaced by collagen fibrils as fibroblasts/myofibroblasts emerge in the interstitial space and alveolar lumen.

Changes occurring during the fibrotic phase include myointimal thickening and mural fibrosis of vessels, which may contribute to the degree of pulmonary hypertension seen in this condition. More strikingly, lung collagen is deposited, the severity of which correlates with an increase in mortality. Although it was once thought that the

Ventilator-Induced Lung Injury

Ventilator Associated Pneumonia

Exudative/Inflammatory Features	Proliferative Features	Fibrotic Features
Epithelial/Endothelial Barrier Dysruption	Destruction of Microvasculature	Myointimal Thickening
Alveolar Wall Oedema	Type II Cell Proliferation (repair)	Mature Fibrosis
Fibrinous Hyaline Membranes	Myofibroblast Proliferation	Cellular Influx
Neutrophil Accumulation	Matrix Production and Fibrosis	Severe Architectural Disruption

OVERLAP

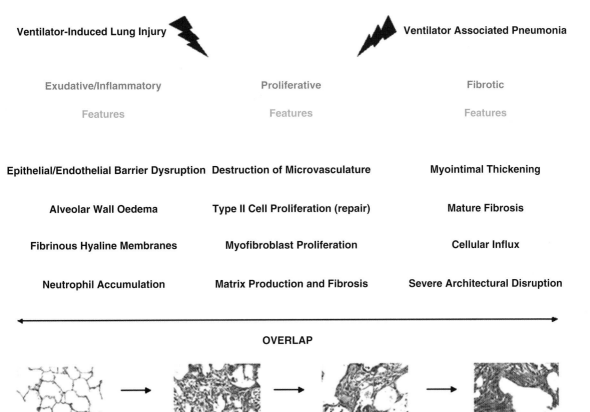

FIGURE 1.1. The pathogenesis of ALI/ARDS.

three phases of ALI/ARDS were distinct and developed sequentially as the condition progressed, there is increasing evidence that there is much overlap between them and, in particular, that the fibrotic phase may be initiated within the first 24 h after diagnosis [8–10].

The cell type predominantly responsible for driving the inflammatory changes in ALI/ARDS is the neutrophil and, predictably, the fibroblast/myofibroblast is the major cell involved in the fibroproliferative phase. A plethora of pro-inflammatory and pro-fibrotic cytokines, chemokines and growth factors are released from resident and recruited cells in ALI/ARDS, which dramatically influence the progression of the condition. In addition, a prevailing procoagulant environment, driven by production of coagulation proteases such as thrombin and factor Xa, oxidant stress and anti-apoptotic factors also play a critical role in orchestrating the response to lung injury. These processes are counterbalanced by regulatory factors which predominately affect resolution of the condition.

ALI/ARDS can also be exacerbated by mechanical ventilation and nosocomial infection leading to ventilator-induced lung injury (VILI) and ventilator-associated pneumonia (VAP), respectively. Although VAP is extremely important to diagnose and treat in patients with ALI/ARDS, the emergence of VILI as an important factor in the progression of this condition has prompted a number of investigators to investigate a mode of ventilation that is 'lung-protective', which will be discussed below. Multifactorial events influence VILI including the induction of shear stresses on alveoli as a result of over-distension and also cyclical opening and closing of atelectatic areas during mechanical ventilation. These events have been

TABLE 1.3. Diagnostic criteria in ALI/ARDS

	Acute lung injury	Acute respiratory distress syndrome
Chest x-ray	Bilateral infiltrates	Bilateral infiltrates
Clinical scenario	Acute onset	Acute onset
Pulmonary artery occlusion pressure	<18 mmHg	<18 mmHg
Oxygenation	PaO_2/FiO_2 ratio <300 mmHg	PaO_2/FiO_2 ratio <200 mmHg

shown to correlate with increased production of pro-inflammatory and pro-fibrotic cytokines. It is also suggested that ALI/ARDS due to VILI can occur in normal lungs if overzealous ventilation is used [11].

Diagnosis

The current American/European definition of ALI/ARDS (Table 1.3) provokes much controversy among intensivists. Protagonists of the definition argue that it is useful as it recognises that severity of lung injury is variable, thereby classifying ALI and ARDS differently, that it is simple and it allows easy comparison of patients across clinical trials. Critics argue that the definition is too simple as it does not take into account the underlying cause. Further criticisms are that the severity of hypox-aemia cut-offs are arbitrary, that individual inter-pretation of the chest x-ray can lead to bias and that current ventilatory strategies, which will be discussed below, are not included in the definition. Finally, although the clinical definition attempts to limit the lung pathology to DAD in the exudative/fibroproliferative phase of ALI/ARDS, other lung pathologies, which have a different pathogenesis, become included when the current diagnostic strategy is used.

Therapeutic Options

Ventilatory Strategies

Tidal Volume

Historically, patients with ALI/ARDS were venti-lated with tidal volumes of 10–15 ml/kg. Due to concerns about VILI in ALI/ARDS a landmark

study examined the effect of reducing tidal volumes to 4–6 mL/kg lean body weight and setting inspiratory plateau pressures (P_{PLAT}) at a maximum of 30 cm of water, in a heterogeneous population with this condition [12]. The study showed that the lower tidal volume group had improved survival (31% vs 40%). It remains con-troversial whether *all* patients with ALI/ARDS should receive low tidal volume ventilation and some investigators advocate that tidal volumes in ALI/ARDS should be based on markers of lung injury that affect respiratory mechanics [13]. A further study appeared to confirm the findings of the ARDSNet study as it showed a significant sur-vival benefit in a heterogeneous group of patients with ALI/ARDS who received lung-protective ventilation compared with patients receiving routine care. However, the results have been greeted with a certain amount of scepticism as the control group in this study were 'historical', had higher Acute Physiology and Chronic Health Evaluation (APACHE) II scores and had a mortal-ity rate of 52%, which is somewhat higher than some recent studies [14]. This problem has been investigated further by re-evaluation of the mor-tality rate of the non-eligible patients from the original ARDSNet trial, under the Freedom of Information Act [15]. Interestingly, they found that low tidal volume ventilation was beneficial in patients whose lungs were less compliant, but patients with more compliant lungs tolerated low tidal volumes poorly, suggesting that a propor-tion of patients may be better managed with tidal volumes >6 mL/kg. Other investigators have sug-gested that using levels of P_{PLAT} described in the ARDSNet study may be a better target than tidal volume for lung-protective ventilation as some patients will reach this level before a tidal volume of 6 mL/kg is achieved [16]. It has also been sug-gested that low tidal volume ventilation may require increased level of sedation and may gen-erate increased levels of intrinsic positive-end expiratory pressure (PEEP) but two recent trials appear to have refuted this [17, 18]. In summary, current evidence supports a low tidal volume, pressure-limited strategy for lung-protective ven-tilation in ALI/ARDS and although the *exact* levels are still under debate, we should use a target of 6 mL/kg lean body weight until better data are available (Figure 1.2).

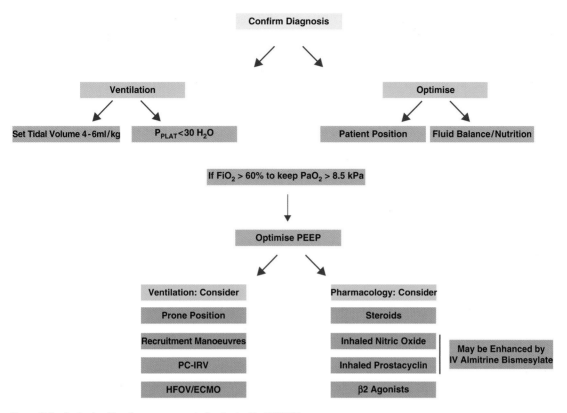

FIGURE 1.2. Basic algorithm for management of patient with ALI/ARDS.

Positive-End Expiratory Pressure (PEEP)

Ashbaugh first noticed that PEEP had beneficial therapeutic effects in ARDS in 1967. PEEP improves gas exchange and pulmonary function in a number of ways. It increases the functional residual capacity, thereby recruiting collapsed alveoli, improving oxygenation and increasing lung compliance. By keeping alveoli open throughout the respiratory cycle, shear forces are reduced, therefore limiting VILI. It also redistributes extravascular lung water and improves ventilation–perfusion matching. Detrimental effects of PEEP also occur including reducing cardiac output and cerebral perfusion and over-distension of areas of less affected lung (reviewed in [19]).

In animal models of lung injury, ventilation with zero PEEP dramatically increases mortality. Despite its favourable effect on oxygenation in animal models and in man, trials have not conclusively demonstrated the effect of PEEP on the outcome of ALI/ARDS or the optimal level for its use in this condition. An ARDSNet randomised controlled trial (RCT) assessed the efficacy of PEEP in ALI/ARDS by comparing a low with a high level [20], but outcome was similar in both groups. Although the question posed was extremely relevant, the study design was criticised, as many investigators believe that setting a universal level of PEEP in all patients with ALI/ARDS was naive and the level should be set on an individual level based on lung mechanics.

Extrapolation from the lung pressure–volume curve was believed to represent the most accurate way to use lung mechanics to set PEEP, with levels set above the lower inflection zone and upper pressure limit set below the upper inflection zone. However, more recently, it has become increasingly apparent that the lung does not operate over a single pressure–volume curve and that affected and unaffected alveoli function differently. The net effect of this is that a level of PEEP that keeps some regions open can lead to over-distension in others.

Two further trials have examined the correct level of PEEP in ALI/ARDS in more detail.

The Express trial, a prospective RCT in 37 French ICUs recruited patients with PF ratios <300 receiving low tidal volume ventilation and randomised them to a 'Minimal distension' group (PEEP 5–9 cmH$_2$O) or a 'Maximal recruitment' group (PEEP increased to achieve plateau pressure 28–30 cmH$_2$O) [21]. The study showed that oxygenation improved and ventilator-free/organ-supported days increased in the high PEEP group. However, there was no change in primary or secondary endpoints of death at 28 and 60 days, respectively. Subgroup analysis showed that in patients who were most hypoxic at the start of the trial, mortality improved in the high PEEP group. These data support the notion that high PEEP should be used in targeted groups.

The Canadian Lung Open Ventilation Trial (LOVE) trial [22] used a control group who received low tidal volume ventilation, plateau airway pressures not exceeding 30 cmH$_2$O with *conventional* levels of PEEP and compared this to an experimental group who received low tidal volume ventilation, plateau pressures not exceeding 40 cmH$_2$O, recruitment manoeuvres and *higher* PEEP. The study showed that the experimental group developed less refractory hypoxaemia and had less 'rescue' therapies but there was no change in the primary or secondary endpoints which were hospital mortality and duration of mechanical ventilation, respectively.

The overall conclusion from these studies is that there is still no real consensus on how lung mechanics can be used to set the ideal PEEP or what the ideal PEEP level is in ALI/ARDS. Although the benefit of PEEP in ALI/ARDS is undoubted, a consensus on the *exact* level required remains undecided.

Recruitment Manoeuvres

Recruitment manoeuvres have been proposed as an adjunct to mechanical ventilation in ALI/ARDS as they have been shown in studies to reduce lung atelectasis, improve oxygenation, prevent endotracheal tube suctioning-induced alveolar derecruitment and derecruitment-associated lung injury and also, together with the application of PEEP, keep newly recruited lung units open (reviewed in [23]). Conversely, other studies have reported them as ineffective, short-acting and dangerous. There are a number of different ways in which they can be done ranging from short-acting bursts of increased PEEP, that is, 40 cm water for 40 s, to complex stepwise alterations of ventilatory pressure. It is thought that recruitment manoeuvres may be more beneficial in extrapulmonary ARDS and if used earlier in the course of the condition.

The most recent trial in this area [24] examined the effect of PEEP recruitment in 67 patients and used whole lung CT to assess its effect. In this study, patients who had the most recruitable lungs had worse survival. This has raised the question as to whether the recruitable lung is in fact the *injured* lung and a marker of disease severity.

This topic remains controversial and, although potentially beneficial, the exact role of recruitment manoeuvres in ALI/ARDS is not yet known and at present it is suggested that they are not used routinely and are reserved for cases of refractory hypoxaemia [25].

Prone Position

Prone positioning has been proposed as a beneficial manoeuvre in ALI/ARDS. The basic rationale behind the strategy is to recruit areas of previously collapsed lung, allowing more homogeneous ventilation, therefore preventing over-distension and VILI. However, a prone-positioned patient generates a number of problems such as potential endotracheal tube displacement, abnormal pressure areas, difficulty in providing adequate cardiopulmonary resuscitation (CPR), difficulty in feeding and the labour-intensive nature of the procedure.

Prone positioning has been shown to improve oxygenation in patients with ALI/ARDS in all studies conducted to date and this is particularly prominent in the early phase of the condition [26]. The favourable effect of the prone position on oxygenation has been confirmed in a recent trial, which also demonstrated that pronation with PEEP-optimisation may reduce VILI [27]. Despite these findings, a large RCT revealed that the prone position does not translate into a survival benefit in ALI/ARDS, although when the most severely hypoxaemic patients in this trial were re-evaluated, there was a trend towards improvement [28]. Another study of prone positioning in hypoxaemic respiratory failure also failed to show reduced mortality, but the proned patients did have a reduced incidence of VAP [29]. A third RCT has also failed to show a mortality benefit [30]. Given the evidence presented above, many ICUs reserve this manoeuvre as a rescue treatment for severely hypoxaemic patients with ALI/ARDS. An ongoing study on this topic by Gattinoni and colleagues will hopefully provide more information on the role of this intervention in ALI/ARDS.

Other Modalities of Ventilation

- Pressure Controlled Inverse Ratio Ventilation (PC-IRV)

The exact mechanisms by which PC-IRV leads to improved gas exchange in ALI/ARDS are not clear but potential advantages are that a longer period of the respiratory cycle is spent at P_{PLAT}, promoting a more homogeneous ventilation pattern, and peak airway pressures are reduced. It is also thought that a benefit may be provided by the shortened expiratory time in PC-IRV, which increases intrinsic PEEP, allowing alveolar compartments which expire slowly to remain open. However, this may also produce dynamic hyperinflation, barotrauma and hypotension, which is undesirable. This mode of ventilation has successfully improved oxygenation when used in ALI/ARDS [31] but its role continues as a rescue therapy at present.

- Airway Pressure Release Ventilation (APRV)

APRV is a form of biphasic positive airways pressure (BIPAP) ventilation that applies two different levels of continuous positive airways pressure (CPAP) with an intermittent pressure release phase. The duration of the lower pressure is short so that the patient breathes at the higher CPAP level. The principle of APRV is that the brief interruption in airway pressure augments spontaneous minute ventilation, which may reduce harmful over-distension of the lung and also improve recruitment. In addition, as breathing is spontaneous in this mode, diaphragmatic and intercostal muscle function is maintained. APRV may provide improved 'open-lung ventilation' but this has yet to be clearly demonstrated in ALI/ARDS.

- High Frequency Oscillation Ventilation (HFOV)

HFOV was first conceived as a potential ventilatory strategy after it was noted that panting dogs take breaths smaller than their dead space, but still maintain oxygenation. The mechanism of this observation is still unknown but it is thought that the high frequency of panting increases turbulence and thus mixing and diffusion of oxygen. This principle is utilised in HFOV, and has had some success as a ventilatory strategy in ALI/ARDS. A small RCT comparing HFOV with a pressure-control ventilatory strategy showed significant improvement in oxygenation at 16h, but neither was this effect prolonged, nor did it improve survival [32]. A more recent study confirmed that the technique is safe and that, when combined with specific recruitment manoeuvres, it caused rapid and sustained improvement in oxygenation [33].

It is hypothesised that the very small tidal volumes, high frequency and constant peak airway pressure used in HFOV may reduce over-distension and VILI and thus have a protective effect in ALI/ARDS. Two large trials, the UK-based OSCAR and Canadian-based OSCILLATE studies, are currently recruiting patients and will attempt to confirm the exact role of HFOV in this condition.

- Extracorporeal Membrane Oxygenation (ECMO) and Partial Liquid Ventilation (PLV)

ECMO is an experimental form of gas exchange which has not yet been shown to be beneficial in ALI/ARDS in clinical trials. However, the technique has been modified recently and complications such as bleeding are fewer. Subsequently, there has been renewed interest in its potential use in this condition. The preliminary results of the Conventional Ventilation or ECMO for Severe Adult Respiratory Failure (CESAR) trial have been announced (but are currently not published) and show that ECMO does appear to improve mortality in ALI/ARDS. However, there are concerns that the results may not be pertinent to all ICUs as the intervention group were all treated in a single centre. The impact of the results of this important trial will be of great interest.

Extracorporeal CO_2 removal is an allied but more limited approach where the main function of the extracorporeal circuit is simply for CO_2 removal, requiring less pressure and lower flow. This technique is not new and was described in the 1980s by Gattinoni in a *Lancet* publication. However, smaller lighter kits have rekindled interest but these all remain experimental at this stage.

PLV is performed by delivering tidal volumes to a perfluorocarbon-treated lung, and the volume of perfluorocarbon instilled is equivalent to that of the functional residual capacity. Preliminary studies in ALI/ARDS have shown that gas exchange and lung mechanics may improve with this approach [35] but complications such as mucus plugging and pneumothoraces may also occur. Again this approach remains only experimental at this stage.

Complications of Ventilating the Patient with ALI/ARDS

In addition to VILI, a number of other complications occur when ventilating the patient with ALI/ARDS. As mentioned above, nosocomial infection can have devastating effects in this condition. However, the diagnosis of VAP, which has a mortality rate of 50% in some studies [36], is a difficult one to make with certainty in patients with ALI/ARDS. The clinical features such as fever, leucocytosis and infiltrates are often similar to the underlying condition and tracheobronchial colonisation clouds the issue microbiologically. Of note, nursing patients in the 45° semi-recumbent position has been shown to decrease VAP [37] and is a simple manoeuvre that should be widely adopted. There is also evidence that continuous aspiration of subglottic secretions (CASS) may prevent VAP [38], but a recent animal study suggests that caution should be exercised with this technique as extensive tracheal mucosal/submucosal damage can occur [39].

Very recent advice from The National Institute for Health and Clinical Excellence (NICE) supports the use of chlorhexidine mouthwashes and raising the head of the bed. Furthermore, a recent trial of silver-coated endotracheal tubes also showed a reduction in the incidence of VAP. However, this study also showed there were no statistically significant between-group differences observed in duration of intubation, intensive care unit stay, hospital stay or mortality, so the impact of this intervention remains to be seen [40].

Pneumothorax is a well-described and potentially fatal complication of ventilating patients with ALI/ARDS, and occurs in 30–87% of subjects depending on the severity of their disease [41]. The radiological and clinical signs may be subtle and quite different to those in patients who are negatively pressure-ventilated and not supine. Small pneumothoraces have the ability to cause catastrophic haemodynamic compromise if untreated, as positive pressure ventilation makes them prone to tensioning. Treatment options include tube thoracostomy, open thoracotomy and image-guided percutaneous catheters; often multiple chest drains are required.

Finally, it has been also been suggested that mechanical ventilation may aggravate acute renal failure via a number of mechanisms including permissive hypercapnia and hypoxia, due to a reduction of renal perfusion as a consequence of reduced cardiac output and also due to 'biotrauma', where pulmonary inflammatory mediators released during ventilation spill over into the systemic circulation. Since all of these processes are exacerbated in ALI/ARDS, the potential for causing renal dysfunction is increased [42].

Pharmacological Agents

Steroids

Steroids are a most plausible treatment option for patients with ALI/ARDS as they possess both anti-inflammatory and anti-fibrotic properties. However, one of the most controversial issues in recent years in ALI/ARDS is whether or not they should be used as a treatment option.

Initial trials of steroids in ALI/ARDS were designed to give short-term, high doses early in the disease, e.g. methyl prednisolone 30 mg/kg 6 hrly for 24 hrs. However, these studies failed to show any benefit and appeared to be associated with increased complications [43, 44] and higher mortality [45]. Other studies have subsequently concentrated on giving steroids for late-phase ARDS. A relatively small study using a lower and more prolonged dose of intravenous methyprednisolone (2 mg/kg loading, then 2 mg/kg in four divided doses, reduced weekly in a tapering fashion), in patients 7 days into 'unresolving' ALI/ARDS, showed that steroid therapy was associated with improved oxygenation and successful extubation [46]. Although this study was promising, its size precluded assumptions on mortality benefit.

In order to resolve this issue, the North American Late Steroid Rescue Study (LaSRS) was conducted by the ARDSNet group and the results recently published [47]. Patients receiving intravenous methylprednisolone had early physiologic and clinical benefits, as they displayed improved oxygenation, lung compliance and came off the ventilator sooner. However, there was no difference in mortality at 60 and 180 days compared with the control group. However, subgroup analysis showed that if bronchoalveolar fluid (BALF) procollagen III peptide levels were high at enrolment into the study, there was a survival benefit with steroids. Interestingly, in this study there was no evidence that steroids increased nosocomial infection but they appeared to increase critical illness polyneuropathy and hypergylcaemia. In summary, there appears to be little evidence to support the routine of steroids in ALI/ARDS but they may have a role in selected patients with a confirmed fibrotic phenotype.

Surfactant

Surfactant is a complex biologic substance made of 90% lipid and 10% protein. The lipid component, mainly dipalmitoylphosphatidylcholine (DPCC), and the protein element are both synthesised and recycled by Type II alveolar epithelial cells. Four individual surfactant proteins exist (SP-A, -B, -C, -D), which enhance surface tension properties and also provide a defence against pathogens.

As briefly discussed above, surfactant levels are severely depleted in ALI/ARDS as Type II epithelial cells are damaged. In addition, the residual surfactant produced is both diluted and inactivated by the florid, proteolytic oedema fluid produced in this condition. For this reason, trying to replace surfactant in patients with ALI/ARDS in clinical trials is arguably one of the more logical pharmacological therapies that has been attempted to date.

A number of trials have used various surfactant preparations, administration regimens and delivery techniques, including aerosolisation in ventilator gas, intratracheal delivery and direct bron-choscopic instillation. These studies have shown that surfactant improved oxygenation in ALI/ARDS,

but none, including the most recent publication which used four intratracheal instillations of lipid and recombinant SP-C over a 24-h period, has shown a survival benefit [48]. However, a post-hoc analysis of the data in this trial suggested that patients with direct ARDS (especially those with severe injury) had reduced mortality.

Various other issues surrounding the potential use of surfactant in ALI/ARDS still need to be resolved including a further understanding of the metabolism and functional impact of exogenous surfactant, the mode, volume and timing of administration and also patient selection. Sadly, a further trial of surfactant in ALI/ARDS with severe primary pulmonary injury has ceased recruitment and there are no current trials of this therapy. However, many still believe that surfactant is still a viable therapy for ALI/ARDS and if biophysical/pharmacological issues surrounding compound preparation can be overcome, it may yet make an impact.

Nitric Oxide

Nitric Oxide (NO) is constitutively produced in the lung but when delivered exogenously in ALI/ARDS augments hypoxic pulmonary vasoconstriction by selectively vasodilating vessels associated with ventilated alveoli. It has also been shown to have favourable effects on pulmonary capillary pressure [49] and pulmonary transvascular albumin flux [50]. The net effect of these events is that ventilation/perfusion matching and oxygenation are improved.

To date there have been three multicentre RCTs assessing the effect of NO in ALI/ARDS [51–53]. In all of these trials, patients receiving NO initially improved oxygenation but this was neither prolonged nor translated into a survival benefit. Although it is suggested that inhaled NO is usually maximally effective at 10 ppm, critics of the RCTs performed to date argue that the dosing regimens used may have led to toxic effects of NO, therefore negating any potential therapeutic benefit.

A recent systematic review by Adhikari and colleagues [54] assessed the impact of inhaled NO on physiological outcomes, morbidity and mortality in ALI/ARDS. Consistent with the results of the various RCTs, they found that NO resulted in a limited improvement in oxygenation but did not reduce mortality (risk ratio 1.10; 95% confidence interval 0.94 to 1.30), the duration of ventilation or the number of days free of ventilation.

Subsequently, controversy remains over whether or not NO is a useful therapeutic option for patients with ALI/ARDS. At present, most intensivists do not advocate the routine use of NO in ALI/ARDS and only use it as rescue therapy. In addition, NO is now only available through a single company and is very expensive. However, a number of studies have begun to look at using NO in combination with other ventilatory modalities such as prone positioning and HFOV [55]. Combination therapies have shown further improvement in oxygenation and are safe, but further RCTs need to be performed to assess the therapeutic role of this strategy in ALI/ARDS. Nebulised prostacyclin (PGI$_2$) and alprostadil (prostaglandin E$_1$) have also been used as alternatives to NO with some success. The combination of NO or PGI$_2$ with intravenous almitrine bismesylate (which enhances hypoxic pulmonary vasoconstriction) may also provide additional benefit.

Finally, it is worthwhile emphasising that although the major clinical trials described in the paragraphs above using surfactant, NO, PEEP and prone position have all led to improvements in oxygenation, this has not been translated into improved outcome, suggesting that oxygenation may not be a useful surrogate measure. It is also possible that high levels of oxygenation are not beneficial; indeed a recent study in a mouse model of acute lung injury suggested better outcomes with moderate hypoxia rather than hyperoxia. The logic behind this is that hypoxia leads to the local pulmonary release of adenosine, which is anti-inflammatory and capable of blocking a number of downstream cellular responses. Perhaps we should aim for 90–92% oxygen saturations and be as worried when the oxygen saturations are 100% as when they are <90%.

Other Pharmacological Agents

A number of other pharmacological agents have been used in clinical trials in ALI/ARDS with limited success and the results of these studies were recently evaluated in a Cochrane Review [56]. Intravenous pulmonary vasodilators (e.g. prostaglandin E$_1$), antioxidants (e.g. N-acetylcysteine) and thromboxane synthase/5-lipoxygenase inhibitors (e.g.

ketoconazole) have displayed some promise but no mortality benefit in trials. A trial of the anti-inflammatory phosphatidic acid inhibitor pentoxifylline showed that 1 month mortality was reduced in patients with ALI/ARDS and metastatic cancer [57], but a larger study in patients with ALI/ARDS alone, using lisofylline, was stopped at the first interim analysis, as a pre-specified level of improvement in the treatment arm was not met [58].

Studies using granulocyte macrophage colony-stimulating factor (GM-CSF) have shown promise for restoring alveolar capillary barrier integrity. Furthermore, there is much current interest in the therapeutic role of β$_2$ agonists in ALI/ARDS, which are thought to tip the balance in favour of alveolar fluid clearance, by stimulating apical sodium and chloride channels in alveolar epithelial cells. They may also exert favourable effects on inflammation and coagulant balance.

The Beta Agonists Lung Injury Study (BALTI) showed that a continuous intravenous infusion of salbutamol (15 µg/kg/h for 7 days) reduced extravascular lung water in ALI/ARDS [59]. The results of future Phase III studies using nebulised/intravenous β$_2$ agonists in ALI/ARDS are awaited with interest. The UK-based MRC funded BALTI-2 study and ARDSNet ALTA trial have begun recruitment.

There is also much current interest in the role of anticoagulants in ALI/ARDS as there is increasing evidence that excessive activation of the coagulation cascade, with the resultant generation of coagulation proteases, plays a central role in driving the inflammatory and fibroproliferative events that occur in this condition. Consistent with this concept, extravascular intra-alveolar accumulation of fibrin and excessive procoagulant activity are found in the lung in ALI/ARDS. Procoagulant activity is promoted in ALI/ARDS as there is a deficiency of anticoagulant factors such as antithrombin III (AT-III) and an abundance of procoagulant factors such as tissue factor/factor VII–VIIa complexes, which can activate factor X, and trigger activation of the coagulation cascade with a resultant generation of thrombin.

In addition to playing a vital role in blood coagulation, thrombin also exerts a plethora of proinflammatory and pro-fibrotic cellular effects in vitro, many of which are mediated via proteolytic activation of the major thrombin receptor, protease-activated receptor (PAR-1). Broncho-alveolar lavage fluid (BALF) thrombin levels are increased in an animal model of ALI/ARDS and studies have shown that direct pharmacological inhibition of thrombin is protective in this model [60]. Furthermore, this effect is even greater when transgenic knockout mice, deficient in PAR-1, are used in this model [61]. These observations suggest that modulation of the coagulation cascade, and more specifically, PAR-1-mediated effects of thrombin, warrant further evaluation as potential therapeutic strategies for the treatment of ALI/ARDS.

A number of anticoagulant agents, such as tissue factor pathway inhibitor (TFPI), site-inactivated factor VIIa, heparin and activated protein C (APC) have shown promise in animal models of ALI/ARDS, but successful clinical trials using these agents have yet to be described. Studies are now underway looking at the effect of APC in ALI/ARDS after it was successfully used in adults with severe sepsis to reduce mortality (PROWESS) [62]. A recent Phase II study of APC in ALI/ARDS by Michael Matthay's group was presented at the American Thoracic Society Congress [63], but the study did not show a mortality benefit. However, the drug was used in the patient group identified as *not* having a survival benefit in post-PROWESS studies. A subgroup of the forthcoming PROW-ESS-Shock trial, which will re-examine the effect of APC in severe sepsis, will also examine whether APC has a role in ALI/ARDS, and the results of this study are awaited with interest.

It is also worth acknowledging that the potential risk of bleeding complications observed in the PROWESS study makes use of direct thrombin inhibitors or other anticoagulants in ALI/ARDS problematic. For this reason, strategies aimed at blocking PAR-1 may yet provide a unique opportunity for selectively interfering with the pro-fibrotic and pro-inflammatory effects of the coagulation cascade in ALI/ARDS, whilst avoiding potential haemostatic complications of blocking coagulation proteases, such as thrombin.

Understanding the role of anticoagulants in ALI/ARDS is a good example of where dramatic advances in basic science have been translated into the clinical arena. Numerous other plausible therapeutic targets have been identified and are currently under intense investigation. For example, a clinical trial of CD-73 modulation in ALI/ARDS

is about to begin. It is hoped that studies such as this will continue to rapidly emerge so that further understanding of the pathogenesis of ALI/ARDS and generation of new therapeutic targets occurs.

Supporting the Patient with ALI/ARDS

Fluid Management and Blood Transfusion

The dramatic and complex inflammatory sequelae that occur in patients with ALI/ARDS often manifest as cardiovascular dysfunction, which leads to poor tissue and organ perfusion. Right ventricular failure can occur as a consequence of pulmonary hypertension which can affect outcome. Severe sepsis also leads to systemic vasodilatation, hypotension and left ventricular dysfunction. Careful management of intravenous fluid administration is clearly part of standard management in ALI/ARDS and the general consensus is that fluids should be administered appropriately to counteract these events, without leading to volume overload. However, in reality this is difficult to achieve and over-zealous administration of fluid often leads to an increase in extravascular lung water and pulmonary oedema, which may be unavoidable when appropriate organ perfusion is being sought.

Invasive monitoring using pulmonary artery (PA) catheters to guide fluid therapy has been a very controversial topic amongst intensivists for some time. However, an ARDSNet study has now shown that the PA catheter should not be routinely used (ARDSNet, 2006). In conjunction with this study the FACTT ARDSNet study examined the effect of a liberal versus conservative fluid management strategy for 7 days (following initial resuscitation), in an attempt to answer this highly debated topic accurately. The study enrolled 1,000 patients to the two groups and had a primary end point of death at 60 days and secondary end points of ventilator-free days, organ failure and lung physiology. There was no change in the primary end point but the conservative fluid therapy group had improved lung function and shortened duration of mechanical ventilation. In addition, there was no increase in shock or renal failure in the conservative group. A pragmatic interpretation of these results is that once the initial resuscitation period (up to 72 h) has passed, patients with ALI/ARDS should have a fluid balance of neutral to –500 mls daily.

The role of blood transfusion in critical care patients has been topical since a study showed that a restrictive strategy for red cell transfusion appeared at least as effective as a liberal strategy when mortality was assessed [66]. Blood transfusion is associated with transfusion-related lung injury (TRALI) and a recent observational cohort study investigated the effect of red cell transfusion in patients with ALI/ARDS. The study found that transfusion in patients with ALI/ARDS was associated with an increase in mortality [67], and a RCT to answer this question definitively is required.

Nutrition

Adequate nutritional support is vital in patients with ALI/ARDS and the enteral route is the most preferable as it has been shown to reduce the incidence of Gram-negative bacterial colonisation and stress ulceration. There has been interest in enteral immunonutrition in ALI/ARDS after a study showed that a low carbohydrate, high-fat formula rich in fish, borage oils and antioxidants reduced pulmonary neutrophil recruitment, improved oxygenation and shortened the length of mechanical ventilation [68]. However, the study failed to show a difference in mortality of the treatment group and a meta-analysis of enteral immunonutrition in ALI/ARDS also failed to show a benefit [69]. A new ARDNet study of omega-3 and antioxidant supplementation versus full feeding has begun and results are awaited.

Radiology

Chest x-rays are part of the diagnosis of ALI/ARDS but are subject to inter-observer variability. Chest computerised tomography (CT) can be very helpful in routine assessment of the patient with ALI/ARDS, is often used to diagnose presence of pneumothoraces and is also useful for showing the effects of VILI in survivors of ALI/ARDS. An unpredicted consequence of the use of chest CT in this condition has been the evolution of the 'baby lung' hypothesis, which has revealed that in most patients with ALI/ARDS, the normally aerated lung has the dimensions of a young child. The concept of 'baby lung' has helped explain VILI in ALI/ARDS and current theories suggest that the smaller the 'baby lung', the greater is the potential for unsafe ventilation [70]. Chest CT has also been used to set PEEP and there is emerging evidence

that electrical impedance tomography may play a role in this field (reviewed by [71]).

Although chest x-rays and CT may be useful in monitoring progression of ALI/ARDS and detecting complications, they are not accurate at differentiating between other conditions that mimic ALI/ARDS radiologically, but may have entirely different treatment protocols. This brings into question the role of the surgical open-lung biopsy in the diagnosis of this condition. On the whole, this technique is avoided as there are fears about risk/benefit of this potentially injurious procedure. Challenging this dogma is a study in selected patients with ALI/ARDS suggesting that open-lung biopsy can be safely performed, often reveals an unsuspected diagnosis and frequently leads to alteration in therapy [72]. Most clinicians remain unconvinced and the rate of lung biopsy has fallen dramatically over the last 2 decades.

Other Daily Management Issues

The process of care in an ICU is fundamentally important and many units are adopting care bundles to ensure compliance with a range of approaches that have been shown to be beneficial such as **f**eeding, **a**nalgesia, **s**edation-stop, **t**hromboembolic prophylaxis, **h**ead-of-bed elevation, stress **u**lcer prevention and **g**lucose control (FASTHUG) (reviewed in [73]).

Every effort must be made to avoid nosocomial infections such as VAP and line sepsis, as they are associated with an excess mortality. Changes in body position help to facilitate bronchial hygiene, improve oxygenation and avoid pressure sores. There is current interest in kinetic therapy (KT), as the use of this technique, which involves the use of successive postural positioning, has been associated with improved outcomes in patients with ALI/ARDS [74, 75]. However, studies on sufficient patient numbers are awaited.

In ventilator management, it is often necessary to use an appropriate level of sedation to avoid patient–ventilator asynchrony. Use of paralytic agents should be avoided as much as possible, as they may be associated with critical illness polyneuropathy. In addition, daily spontaneous breathing trials are useful in patients weaning from the ventilator in ALI/ARDS and may facilitate earlier extubation.

WEB-LINKS

Topic	Web-link
The Intercollegiate Board for Training in Intensive Care Medicine	http://www.rcoa.ac.uk/ibticm/
Intensive Care Society Website	http://www.ics.ac.uk/
NHLI ARDSNet Website	http://www.ardsnet.org/
NICE Guidelines for use of Activated Protein C in Sepsis	http://www.nice.org.uk/page.aspx?o = 221104
PubMed: National Library of Medicine's Search Service	http://www.ncbi.nlm.nih.gov/entrez/query.fcgi
Education, care, support and communication for patients, survivors, families, friends, medical personnel and others affected by, and/or interested in, ARDS	http://www.ards.org/
CESAR Trial Website	http://www.cesar-trial.org/

Finally, a number of important clinical trials, which are directly pertinent to day-to-day care of patients with ALI/ARDS, are ongoing. The TracMan trial is a good example of such a study, which is examining whether patients predicted to require ventilatory support for 7 days or more, who have a tracheostomy sited on day 1–4 following ICU admission, have a reduced mortality at day 30, compared with a tracheostomy sited on or after day 10.

How Do Survivors Perform?

Surviving an ICU stay with severe ALI/ARDS requires enormous input and cohesion from the multidisciplinary team responsible for patient care. Although discharge of a patient from the ICU after a prolonged stay is extremely rewarding, it is increasingly recognised that long-term disability occurs when survivors are followed up.

Survivors have been reported to have cognitive defects, depression, post-traumatic stress disorder and are often unable to return to employment which undoubtedly has a large morbidity (reviewed in [76]). In addition, lung function in survivors reveals that residual obstructive and restrictive defects are common. Impaired gas exchange is also frequently observed and cardiopulmonary exercise testing is particularly sensitive at detecting this [77].

Although it is well recognised that abnormal pulmonary function and symptoms occur after ALI/ARDS, their relationship to overall health-related quality of life is disputed. Interestingly, significant correlations have been shown to exist between these factors, suggesting that underlying lung injury does correlate with long-term morbidity [76]. Finally, in addition to the problems faced by patients with ALI/ARDS, it is increasingly recognised that spouses, relatives and carers have to carry a large psychological burden in the period of patient convalescence.

References

1. Bernard GR. Acute respiratory distress syndrome: a historical perspective. Am J Respir Crit Care Med. 2005 Oct 1;172(7):798–806. Epub 2005 Jul 14.
2. Bernard GR, Artigas A, Brigham KL, Carlet J, Falke K, Hudson L, Lamy M, Legall JR, Morris A, Spragg R. The American-European Consensus Conference on ARDS. Definitions, mechanisms, relevant outcomes, and clinical trial coordination. Am J Respir Crit Care Med. 1994 Mar;149(3 Pt 1):818–24. Review.
3. Irish Critical Care Trials Group. Acute lung injury and the acute respiratory distress syndrome in Ireland: a prospective audit of epidemiology and management. Crit Care. 2008;12(1):R30. Epub 2008 Feb 29.
4. Rubenfeld GD, Caldwell E, Peabody E, Weaver J, Martin DP, Neff M, Stern EJ, Hudson LD. Incidence and outcomes of acute lung injury. N Engl J Med. 2005 Oct 20;353(16):1685–93.
5. Ware LB, Matthay MA The acute respiratory distress syndrome. N Engl J Med. 2000 May 4;342(18): 1334–49.
6. Marshall RP, Webb S, Bellingan GJ, Montgomery HE, Chaudhari B, McAnulty RJ, Humphries SE, Hill MR, Laurent GJ. Angiotensin converting enzyme insertion/deletion polymorphism is associated with susceptibility and outcome in acute respiratory distress syndrome. Am J Respir Crit Care Med. 2002 Sep 1; 166(5):646–50.
7. Bellingan GJ. The pulmonary physician in critical care * 6: The pathogenesis of ALI/ARDS. Thorax. 2002 Jun;57(6):540–6.

8. Chesnutt AN, Matthay MA, Tibayan FA et al. Early detection of type III procollagen peptide in acute lung injury. Pathogenetic and prognostic significance. Am J Respir Crit Care Med. 1997 Sep;156 (3 Pt 1):840–5.

9. Marshall RP, Bellingan G, Webb S et al. Fibroproliferation occurs early in the acute respiratory distress syndrome and impacts on outcome. Am J Respir Crit Care Med. 2000 Nov;162(5):1783–8.

10. Howell DCJ, Falzon M, Bilbe N, Bottoms SE, Laurent GJ, Bellingan GJ, Chambers RC. Pulmonary fibrosis occurs early in acute lung injury/acute respiratory distress syndrome (ALI/ARDS) and is associated with expression of protease activated receptor-1 (PAR1). Am J Respir Crit Care Med. 2007 May, A950.

11. Gajic O, Dara SI, Mendez JL, Adesanya AO, Festic E, Caples SM, Rana R, St Sauver JL, Lymp JF, Afessa B, Hubmayr RD. Ventilator-associated lung injury in patients without acute lung injury at the onset of mechanical ventilation. Crit Care Med. 2004 Sep;32(9):1817–24.

12. NIH/NHLBI ARDSNet. Ventilation with lower tidal volumes as compared with traditional tidal volumes for acute lung injury and the acute respiratory distress syndrome. New Engl J Med. 2000;342:1301–8.

13. Gattinoni L, Eleonora C, Caironi P. Monitoring of pulmonary mechanics in acute respiratory distress syndrome to titrate therapy. Curr Opin Crit Care. 2005 Jun;11(3):252–8.

14. Kallet RH, Jasmer RM, Pittet JF, Tang JF, Campbell AR, Dicker R, Hemphill C, Luce JM. Clinical implementation of the ARDS network protocol is associated with reduced hospital mortality compared with historical controls. Crit Care Med. 2005 May;33(5):925–9.

15. Deans KJ, Minneci PC, Cui X, Banks SM, Natanson C, Eichacker PQ. Mechanical ventilation in ARDS: One size does not fit all. Crit Care Med. 2005 May;33(5): 1141–3.

16. Eichacker PQ, Gerstenberger EP, Banks SM, Cui X, Natanson C. Meta-analysis of acute lung injury and acute respiratory distress syndrome trials testing low tidal volumes. Am J Respir Crit Care Med. 2002 Dec 1; 166(11):1510–4. Epub 2002 Aug 28.

17. Kahn JM, Andersson L, Karir V, Polissar NL, Neff MJ, Rubenfeld GD. Low tidal volume ventilation does not increase sedation use in patients with acute lung injury. Crit Care Med. 2005 Apr;33(4):766–71.

18. Hough CL, Kallet RH, Ranieri VM, Rubenfeld GD, Luce JM, Hudson LD. Intrinsic positive end-expiratory pressure in acute respiratory distress syndrome (ARDS) Network subjects. Crit Care Med. 2005 Mar;33(3):527–32.

19. Villar J. The use of positive end-expiratory pressure in the management of the acute respiratory distress syndrome. Minerva Anestesiol. 2005 Jun;71(6):265–72.

20. Brower RG, Lanken PN, MacIntyre NR, Matthay MA, Morris AH, Ancukiewicz M, Schoenfeld DA, Thompson BT. NIH/NHLBI ARDSNet. Higher versus lower positive end-expiratory pressures in patients with the acute respiratory distress syndrome. New Engl J Med. 2004 Jul 22;351(4):327–36.

21. Mercat A, Richard JC, Vielle B, Jaber S, Osman D, Diehl JL, Lefrant JY, Prat G, Richecoeur J, Nieszkowska A, Gervais C, Baudot J, Bouadma L, Brochard L. Positive end-expiratory pressure setting in adults with acute lung injury and acute respiratory distress syndrome: a randomized controlled trial. Expiratory Pressure (Express) Study Group. JAMA. 2008 Feb 13; 299(6):646–55.

22. Meade MO, Cook DJ, Guyatt GH, Slutsky AS, Arabi YM, Cooper DJ, Davies AR, Hand LE, Zhou Q, Thabane L, Austin P, Lapinsky S, Baxter A, Russell J, Skrobik Y, Ronco JJ, Stewart TE, Lung Open Ventilation Study Investigators. Ventilation strategy using low tidal volumes, recruitment maneuvers, and high positive end-expiratory pressure for acute lung injury and acute respiratory distress syndrome: a randomized controlled trial. JAMA. 2008 Feb 13;299(6):637–45.

23. Koh WJ, Suh GY, Han J, Lee SH, Kang EH, Chung MP, Kim H, Kwon OJ. Recruitment maneuvers attenuate repeated derecruitment-associated lung injury. Crit Care Med. 2005 May;33(5):1070–6.

24. Gattinoni L, Caironi P, Cressoni M, Chiumello D, Ranieri VM, Quintel M, Russo S, Patroniti N, Cornejo R, Bugedo G. Lung recruitment in patients with the acute respiratory distress syndrome. N Engl J Med. 2006 Apr 27;354(17):1775–86.

25. Caironi P, Gattinoni L. How to monitor lung recruitment in patients with acute lung injury. Curr Opin Crit Care. 2007 Jun;13(3):338–43.

26. Mure M, Domino KB, Lindahl SG, Hlastala MP, Altemeier WA, Glenny RW. Regional ventilation-perfusion distribution is more uniform in the prone position. J Appl Physiol. 2000 Mar;88(3):1076–83.

27. Mentzelopoulos SD, Roussos C, Zakynthinos SG. Prone position reduces lung stress and strain in severe acute respiratory distress syndrome. Eur Respir J. 2005 Mar;25(3):534–44.

28. Gattinoni L, Tognoni G, Pesenti A, Taccone P, Mascheroni D, Labarta V, Malacrida R, Di Giulio P, Fumagalli R, Pelosi P, Brazzi L, Latini R, Prone-Supine Study Group. Effect of prone positioning on the survival of patients with acute respiratory failure. N Engl J Med. 2001 Aug 23;345(8):568–73.

29. Guerin C, Gaillard S, Lemasson S, Ayzac L, Girard R, Beuret P, Palmier B, Le QV, Sirodot M, Rosselli S, Cadiergue V, Sainty JM, Barbe P, Combourieu E, Debatty D, Rouffineau J, Ezingeard E, Millet O, Guelon D, Rodriguez L, Martin O, Renault A, Sibille JP, Kaidomar M. Effects of systematic prone positioning in

hypoxemic acute respiratory failure: a randomized controlled trial. JAMA. 2004 Nov 17;292(19):2379–87.

30. Mancebo J, Fernández R, Blanch L, Rialp G, Gordo F, Ferrer M, Rodríguez F, Garro P, Ricart P, Vallverdú I, Gich I, Castaño J, Saura P, Domínguez G, Bonet A, Albert RK. A multicenter trial of prolonged prone ventilation in severe acute respiratory distress syndrome. Am J Respir Crit Care Med. 2006 Jun 1; 173(11):1233–9. Epub 2006 Mar 23.

31. Wang SH, Wei TS. The outcome of early pressure-controlled inverse ratio ventilation on patients with severe acute respiratory distress syndrome in surgical intensive care unit. Am J Surg. 2002 Feb;183(2):151–5.

32. Derdak S. High-frequency oscillatory ventilation for acute respiratory distress syndrome in adult patients. Crit Care Med. 2003 Apr;31(4 Suppl):S317–23.

33. Ferguson ND, Chiche JD, Kacmarek RM, Hallett DC, Mehta S, Findlay GP, Granton JT, Slutsky AS, Stewart TE. Combining high-frequency oscillatory ventilation and recruitment maneuvers in adults with early acute respiratory distress syndrome: the Treatment with Oscillation and an Open Lung Strategy (TOOLS) Trial pilot study. Crit Care Med. 2005 Mar;33(3):479–86.

34. Gattinoni L, Pesenti A, Bombino M, Pelosi P, Brazzi L. Role of extracorporeal circulation in adult respiratory distress syndrome management. New Horiz. 1993 Nov;1(4):603–12.

35. Hirschl RB, Pranikoff T, Wise C, Overbeck MC, Gauger P, Schreiner RJ, Dechert R, Bartlett RH. Initial experience with partial liquid ventilation in adult patients with the acute respiratory distress syndrome. JAMA. 1996 Feb 7;275(5):383–9.

36. Rello J, Quintana E, Ausina V, Castella J, Luquin M, Net A, Prats G. Incidence, etiology, and outcome of nosocomial pneumonia in mechanically ventilated patients. Chest. 1991 Aug;100(2):439–44.

37. Drakulovic MB, Torres A, Bauer TT, Nicolas JM, Nogué S, Ferrer M. Supine body position as a risk factor for nosocomial pneumonia in mechanically ventilated patients: a randomised trial. Lancet. 1999 Nov 27;354(9193):1851–8.

38. Ewig S, Torres A. Prevention and management of ventilator-associated pneumonia. Curr Opin Crit Care. 2002 Feb;8(1):58–69.

39. Berra L, De Marchi L, Panigada M, Yu ZX, Baccarelli A, Kolobow T. Evaluation of continuous aspiration of subglottic secretion in an in vivo study. Crit Care Med. 2004 Oct;32(10):2071–8.

40. Kollef MH, Afessa B, Anzueto A, Veremakis C, Kerr KM, Margolis BD, Craven DE, Roberts PR, Arroliga AC, Hubmayr RD, Restrepo MI, Auger WR, Schinner R, NASCENT Investigation Group. Silver-coated endotracheal tubes and incidence of ventilator-associated pneumonia: the NASCENT randomized trial. JAMA. 2008 Aug 20;300(7):805–13.

41. Gattinoni L, Bombino M, Pelosi P, Lissoni A, Pesenti A, Fumagalli R, Tagliabue M. Lung structure and function in different stages of severe adult respiratory distress syndrome. JAMA. 1994 Jun 8;271(22):1772–9.

42. Kuiper JW, Groeneveld AB, Slutsky AS, Plötz FB. Mechanical ventilation and acute renal failure. Crit Care Med. 2005 Jun;33(6):1408–15.

43. Bernard GR, Luce JM, Sprung CL, Rinaldo JE, Tate RM, Sibbald WJ, Kariman K, Higgins S, Bradley R, Metz CA, et al. High-dose corticosteroids in patients with the adult respiratory distress syndrome. N Engl J Med. 1987 Dec 17;317(25):1565–70.

44. Luce JM, Montgomery AB, Marks JD, Turner J, Metz CA, Murray JF. Ineffectiveness of high-dose methylprednisolone in preventing parenchymal lung injury and improving mortality in patients with septic shock. Am Rev Respir Dis. 1988 Jul;138(1):62–8.

45. Bone RC, Fisher CJ Jr, Clemmer TP, Slotman GJ, Metz CA. Early methylprednisolone treatment for septic syndrome and the adult respiratory distress syndrome. Chest. 1987 Dec;92(6):1032–6.

46. Meduri GU, Headley AS, Golden E, Carson SJ, Umberger RA, Kelso T, Tolley EA. Effect of prolonged methylprednisolone therapy in unresolving acute respiratory distress syndrome: a randomized controlled trial. JAMA. 1998 Jul 8;280(2):159–65.

47. Steinberg KP, Hudson LD, Goodman RB, Hough CL, Lanken PN, Hyzy R, Thompson BT, Ancukiewicz M, National Heart, Lung, and Blood Institute Acute Respiratory Distress Syndrome (ARDS) Clinical Trials Network. Efficacy and safety of corticosteroids for persistent acute respiratory distress syndrome. N Engl J Med. 2006 Apr 20;354(16):1671–84.

48. Spragg RG, Lewis JF, Walmrath HD, Johannigman J, Bellingan G, Laterre PF, Witte MC, Richards GA, Rippin G, Rathgeb F, Häfner D, Taut FJ, Seeger W. Effect of recombinant surfactant protein C-based surfactant on the acute respiratory distress syndrome. N Engl J Med. 2004 Aug 26;351(9):884–92.

49. Benzing A, Geiger K. Inhaled nitric oxide lowers pulmonary capillary pressure and changes longitudinal distribution of pulmonary vascular resistance in patients with acute lung injury. Acta Anaesthesiol Scand. 1994 Oct;38(7):640–5.

50. Benzing A, Bräutigam P, Geiger K, Loop T, Beyer U, Moser E. Inhaled nitric oxide reduces pulmonary transvascular albumin flux in patients with acute lung injury. Anesthesiology. 1995 Dec; 83(6): 1153–61.

51. Dellinger RP, Zimmerman JL, Taylor RW, Straube RC, Hauser DL, Criner GJ, Davis K Jr, Hyers TM, Papadakos P. Effects of inhaled nitric oxide in patients with acute respiratory distress syndrome: results of a randomized phase II trial. Inhaled Nitric Oxide in ARDS Study Group. Crit Care Med. 1998 Jan;26(1):15–23.

52. Lundin S, Mang H, Smithies M, Stenqvist O, Frostell C. Inhalation of nitric oxide in acute lung injury: results of a European multicentre study. The European Study Group of Inhaled Nitric Oxide. Intensive Care Med. 1999 Sep;25(9):911–9.

53. Taylor RW, Zimmerman JL, Dellinger RP, Straube RC, Criner GJ, Davis K Jr, Kelly KM, Smith TC, Small RJ, Inhaled Nitric Oxide in ARDS Study Group. Low-dose inhaled nitric oxide in patients with acute lung injury: a randomized controlled trial. JAMA. 2004 Apr 7;291(13):1603–9.

54. Adhikari NK, Burns KE, Friedrich JO, Granton JT, Cook DJ, Meade MO. Effect of nitric oxide on oxygenation and mortality in acute lung injury: systematic review and meta-analysis. BMJ. 2007 Apr 14; 334(7597):779. Epub 2007 Mar 23.

55. Fan E, Mehta S. High-frequency oscillatory ventilation and adjunctive therapies: inhaled nitric oxide and prone positioning. Crit Care Med. 2005 Mar;33 (3 Suppl):S182–7.

56. Adhikari N, Burns KE, Meade MO. Pharmacologic therapies for adults with acute lung injury and acute respiratory distress syndrome. Cochrane Database Syst Rev. 2004 Oct 18;(4):CD004477.

57. Ardizzoia A, Lissoni P, Tancini G, Paolorossi F, Crispino S, Villa S, Barni S. Respiratory distress syndrome in patients with advanced cancer treated with pentoxifylline: a randomized study. Support Care Cancer. 1993 Nov;1(6):331–3.

58. [No authors listed] Randomized, placebo-controlled trial of lisofylline for early treatment of acute lung injury and acute respiratory distress syndrome. Crit Care Med. 2002 Jan;30(1):1–6.

59. Perkins GD, McAuley DF, Thickett DR, Gao F. The beta-agonist lung injury trial (BALTI): a randomized placebo-controlled clinical trial. Am J Respir Crit Care Med. 2006 Feb 1;173(3):281–7. Epub 2005 Oct 27.

60. Howell DC, Goldsack NR, Marshall RP, McAnulty RJ, Starke R, Purdy G, Laurent GJ, Chambers RC. Direct thrombin inhibition reduces lung collagen, accumulation, and connective tissue growth factor mRNA levels in bleomycin-induced pulmonary fibrosis. Am J Pathol. 2001 Oct;159(4):1383–95.

61. Howell DC, Johns RH, Lasky JA, Shan B, Scotton CJ, Laurent GJ, Chambers RC. Absence of proteinase-activated receptor-1 signaling affords protection from bleomycin-induced lung inflammation and fibrosis. Am J Pathol. 2005 May;166(5):1353–65.

62. Bernard GR, Vincent JL, Laterre PF, LaRosa SP, Dhainaut JF, Lopez-Rodriguez A, Steingrub JS, Garber GE, Helterbrand JD, Ely EW, Fisher CJ Jr, Recombinant human protein C Worldwide Evaluation in Severe Sepsis (PROWESS) study group. Efficacy and safety of recombinant human activated protein C for severe sepsis. N Engl J Med. 2001 Mar 8; 344(10):699–709.

63. Liu KD, Levitt JH, Zhuo M, et al. Randomized, placebo-controlled trial of activated protein C for the treatment of acute lung injury, [ATS International Conference, Toronto 2008, Publication Page: A766].

64. Wheeler AP, Bernard GR, Thompson BT, Schoenfeld DA, Wiedemann HP, deBoisblanc BP, Connors Jr, AF, Hite RD, Harabin AL, NIH/NHLBI ARDSNet. Pulmonary-artery versus central venous catheter to guide treatment of acute lung injury, New Engl J Med. 2006 May 21; 354(21):2213–24. Epub.

65. Wiedemann HP, Wheeler AP, Bernard GR, Thompson BT, Hayden D, deBoisblanc BP, Connors Jr, AF, Hite RD, Harabin AL, NIH/NHLBI ARDSNet. Comparison of Two Fluid-Management Strategies in Acute Lung Injury, New Engl J Med. 2006 May 21;354(24):2564–75. Epub.

66. Hébert PC, Wells G, Tweeddale M, Martin C, Marshall J, Pham B, Blajchman M, Schweitzer I, Pagliarello G. Does transfusion practice affect mortality in critically ill patients? Transfusion Requirements in Critical Care (TRICC) Investigators and the Canadian Critical Care Trials Group. Am J Respir Crit Care Med. 1997 May;155(5):1618–23.

67. Gong MN, Thompson BT, Williams P, Pothier L, Boyce PD, Christiani DC. Clinical predictors of and mortality in acute respiratory distress syndrome: potential role of red cell transfusion. Crit Care Med. 2005 Jun;33(6):1191–8.

68. Gadek JE, DeMichele SJ, Karlstad MD, Pacht ER, Donahoe M, Albertson TE, Van Hoozen C, Wennberg AK, Nelson JL, Noursalehi M. Effect of enteral feeding with eicosapentaenoic acid, gamma-linolenic acid, and antioxidants in patients with acute respiratory distress syndrome. Enteral Nutrition in ARDS Study Group. Crit Care Med. 1999 Aug;27(8):1409–20.

69. Beale RJ, Bryg DJ, Bihari DJ. Immunonutrition in the critically ill: a systematic review of clinical outcome. Crit Care Med. 1999 Dec;27(12):2799–805.

70. Gattinoni L, Pesenti A. The concept of "baby lung". Intensive Care Med. 2005 Jun;31(6):776–84. Epub 2005 Apr 6.

71. Barbas CS, de Matos GF, Pincelli MP, da Rosa Borges E, Antunes T, de Barros JM, Okamoto V, Borges JB, Amato MB, de Carvalho CR. Mechanical ventilation in acute respiratory failure: recruitment and high positive end-expiratory pressure are necessary. Curr Opin Crit Care. 2005 Feb;11(1):18–28.

72. Patel SR, Karmpaliotis D, Ayas NT, Mark EJ, Wain J, Thompson BT, Malhotra A. The role of open-lung biopsy in ARDS. Chest. 2004 Jan;125(1):197–202.

73. Vincent JL. Give your patient a fast hug (at least) once a day. Crit Care Med. 2005 Jun;33(6):1225–9.

74. Chechenin MG, Voevodin SV, Pronichev EIu, Shuliveĭstrov IuV. Kinetic therapy for acute respiratory distress syndrome. Anesteziol Reanimatol. 2004 Nov–Dec;(6):8–12.

75. Rance M. Kinetic therapy positively influences oxygenation in patients with ALI/ARDS. Nurs Crit Care. 2005 Jan–Feb;10(1):35–41.

76. Heyland DK, Groll D, Caeser M. Survivors of acute respiratory distress syndrome: relationship between pulmonary dysfunction and long-term health-related quality of life. Crit Care Med. 2005 Jul;33(7):1549–56.

77. Neff TA, Stocker R, Frey HR, Stein S, Russi EW. Long-term assessment of lung function in survivors of severe ARDS. Chest. 2003 Mar;123(3):845–53.

2
Life-Threatening Asthma

John E.S. Park and Mark J.D. Griffiths

Abstract Acute severe asthma is a life-threatening condition that, in the majority of cases, has a slow onset and is preventable with early and appropriate treatment. For those who present to hospital, corticosteroids and nebulised β_2-agonists and ipratropium bromide should be administered according to published guidelines. Patients who fail to respond to first-line treatment should be assessed by the intensive care team and placed in an environment where tracheal intubation can be rapidly and safely performed. The object of intensive care management of the critically ill asthma patient is to buy time for medical therapy to work whilst causing minimal harm.

Introduction

Asthma is an inflammatory airway disease characterised by airway hyper-responsiveness and reversible airflow limitation that produces wheezing, shortness of breath and cough. The diagnosis of asthma is based on the history and evidence of reversible airflow limitation.[8] The prevalence in adults varies geographically; 1,600 deaths per year in the UK and 100,000 per year worldwide are attributable to asthma.[1,2] The British Thoracic Society (BTS) has defined grades of asthma severity according to the patient's peak expiratory flow rate (PEFR) (Table 2.1).[8] This review will address the pathophysiology, recognition and management of life-threatening exacerbations of asthma.

Pathophysiology

Both exogenous and endogenous stimuli (e.g. pollen, exercise and infection) may initiate the release of and activation of mediators of inflammation including histamine, leukotrienes and cytokines.[3,4] Narrowing of the bronchial lumen occurs by bronchoconstriction, mucosal thickening related to inflammation and mucus hypersecretion[3,4] (Figure 2.1).

Patients who die from asthma may be divided into two groups. In 80–90%, there is a progressive deterioration over days (type 1 or slow onset acute asthma).[5,6] These patients are more commonly female and infection is often the precipitating factor.[7] Eosinophilic inflammation predominates, mucus plugging is seen and consequently resolution of the attack is slow. Type 2 or sudden asphyxic acute asthma occurs more rapidly over a few hours and accounts for 8–14% of severe asthma exacerbations with a slight male preponderance.[5,6] In this group, allergens, exercise and psychological stress are more common precipitants, although in half the trigger may not be evident.[5,6] Airway obstruction at presentation is generally more severe but response to treatment is quicker than in type 1 severe asthma.[8] Post-mortem studies reveal empty airways consistent with severe bronchospasm, and predominantly neutrophilic inflammation.[9,10]

Airway obstruction disproportionately retards expiratory flow, which coupled with high ventilatory demand and a shortened expiratory time may result in incomplete alveolar emptying and so-called

TABLE 2.1. Definitions of severe and life-threatening asthma

Acute severe asthma	One of: • PEFR 33–50% best predicted • Respiratory rate ≥ 25/min • Heart rate ≥ 110/min • Unable to complete a full sentence
Life-threatening asthma	Severe asthma plus one of • PEFR < 33% best predicted • SpO_2 < 92% • PaO_2 < 8 kPa • Silent chest • Cyanosis • Poor respiratory effort
Near fatal asthma	Raised $PaCO_2$ Requiring mechanical ventilation

Abbreviations: PEFR, peak expiratory flow rate; SpO_2, oxygen saturation measured by pulse oximetry; PaO_2, arterial oxygen partial pressure; $PaCO_2$, arterial partial pressure of carbon dioxide.
Source: Adapted from Annex 4 of the BTS/SIGN Asthma Guidelines.[15]

dynamic hyperinflation (Figure 2.2). Alveolar end-expiratory pressures rise creating intrinsic positive end-expiratory pressure (PEEPi) or auto-PEEP. The diaphragms become flattened reducing their efficiency and an increase in dead space at higher lung volumes requires a rise in minute volume to maintain adequate ventilation.[11] The combination of decreased venous return and increased right ventricular afterload resulting from increased pulmonary vascular resistance causes cardiovascular compromise (Figure 2.1). This may manifest clinically as pulsus paridoxicus or cardiac arrest on initiating positive pressure ventilation.

Arterial blood gas analysis in acute severe asthma commonly reveals hypoxaemia caused by ventilation/perfusion (V/Q) mismatching, with hypocapnia and respiratory alkalosis. In the most severe cases, hypercapnia may develop as a result of muscle fatigue and the inability to maintain adequate alveolar ventilation. Respiratory acidosis accompanies hypercapnia and lactic acidosis may result from increased muscle activity and tissue hypoxia.[12]

Epidemiology and Risk Stratification

Most asthma deaths occur outside hospital.[13] Unsurprisingly, poor compliance and asthma control are markers for increased severity of exacerbations and increasing or heavy use of β_2-agonists increase the risk of fatal or near fatal asthma.[14,15] Females have an overall higher risk for acute severe asthma and adverse behavioural or psychosocial factors also increase the risk of developing severe exacerbations.[7,16] Previous hospital admissions and admissions to ICU are risk factors for developing life-threatening asthma, although their absence does not imply decreased risk (Table 2.2).[7,17,18]

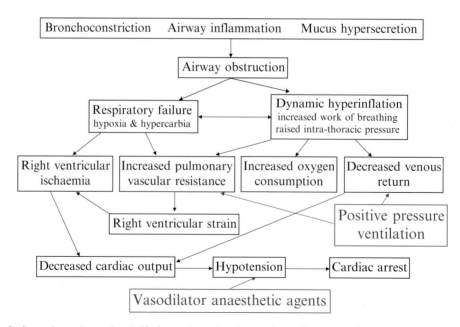

FIGURE 2.1. Cardio-respiratory interactions in life threatening asthma Iatrogenic contributions in red.

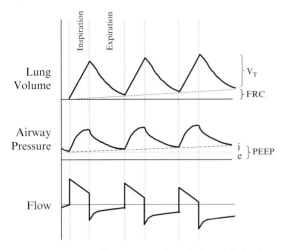

FIGURE 2.2. Diagram demonstrating dynamic hyperinflation in a mechanically ventilated patient with expiratory airflow limitation caused by severe asthma

Dynamic hyperinflation or breath stacking caused by gas trapping occurs when a breath is delivered before expiration of the previous breath has been completed. In this case, the set ratio of inspiration/expiration is 1:2 (normal) but the retarded expiratory flow results in a progressive increase in airway pressure (Paw) and functional residual capacity (FRC). In addition, the positive end-expiratory pressure (PEEP) increases. This is comprised of an extrinsic or set (e) and dynamic intrinsic (i) components. Apart from the expiratory time, the tidal volume and respiratory rate will also determine the extent of breath stacking. V_T — tidal volume.

TABLE 2.2. Risk factors for life-threatening asthma

Asthma history	Adverse behavioural or psychosocial factors
Previous near fatal asthma (including ICU admission, ventilation and/or hypercapnia)	Non-compliance with treatment, monitoring or clinic appointments
Heavy use of β_2-agonist	Previous hospital self-discharge
Repeated attendances to casualty or admissions to hospital within the last year	History of psychiatric illness including deliberate self-harm
Requiring ≥ three types of asthma medication	Alcohol or drug abuse
	Obesity
	Learning difficulties
	Employment and income difficulties
	Social isolation
	Childhood abuse

Source: Adapted from BTS/SIGN Asthma Guidelines.

The use of oral corticosteroids and antibiotics was associated with reduced mortality in a case control study of 532 patients with acute severe asthma, suggesting that early intervention prevents severe exacerbations.[14]

Clinical Assessment and Monitoring

Initial clinical assessment should be accompanied by aggressive treatment when the diagnosis is confirmed. The PEFR at presentation and its response to treatment have prognostic significance. For severe asthma exacerbations, oxygen saturation by pulse oximetry (SpO_2) should be intermittently recorded with the respiratory rate, pulse and blood pressure. It is recommended that arterial blood gas analysis be performed in those with $SpO_2 \leq 92\%$.[15] Hypoxia ($PaO_2 < 8\,kPa$ irrespective of oxygen therapy), a normal or raised $PaCO_2$, and acidosis are suggestive of life-threatening asthma. A chest radiograph should be performed to exclude pneumothorax and pneumonia, although the yield is low.[19] Continuous electrocardiographic monitoring is recommended to identify dysrhythmias secondary to therapy or worsening cardiorespiratory status. The electrocardiograph commonly shows sinus tachycardia with right axis deviation and right ventricular strain.[12] Any patient with a severe exacerbation of asthma should be placed where suitable monitoring is available, for example, in a high dependency unit (HDU) or resuscitation bay in the Accident and Emergency department or medical admissions unit. The intensive care team should assess immediately any patient identified as having life-threatening asthma (Table 2.1).

Treatment

The BTS guidelines recommend correction of hypoxia with high concentrations of inspired oxygen (40–60%) via a high flow mask and the use of oxygen-driven nebulised β-agonist (salbutamol or terbutaline)[15] (Figure 2.3). Corticosteroids are recommended in high doses and can be administered either orally, as prednisolone, or parenterally, as hydrocortisone.[15] Medications worsening airway obstruction, such as β-blockers, aspirin, non-steroidal anti-inflammatory drugs and adenosine, should be stopped (Table 2.3).

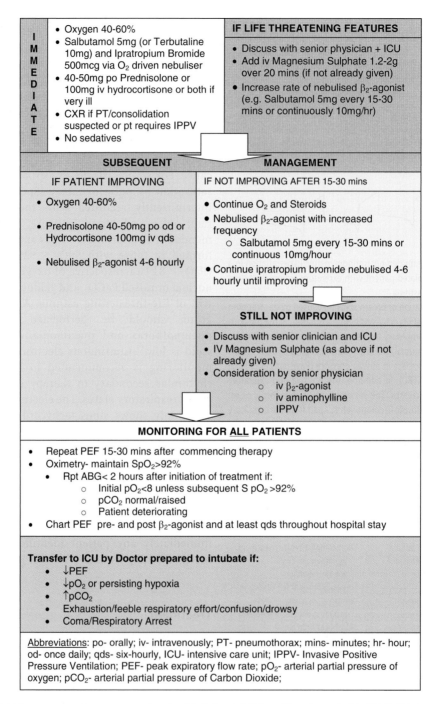

| **IMMEDIATE** | • Oxygen 40-60%
• Salbutamol 5mg (or Terbutaline 10mg) and Ipratropium Bromide 500mcg via O$_2$ driven nebuliser
• 40-50mg po Prednisolone or 100mg iv hydrocortisone or both if very ill
• CXR if PT/consolidation suspected or pt requires IPPV
• No sedatives | **IF LIFE THREATENING FEATURES**

• Discuss with senior physician + ICU
• Add iv Magnesium Sulphate 1.2-2g over 20 mins (if not already given)
• Increase rate of nebulised β$_2$-agonist (e.g. Salbutamol 5mg every 15-30 mins or continuously 10mg/hr) |

SUBSEQUENT	**MANAGEMENT**
IF PATIENT IMPROVING	IF NOT IMPROVING AFTER 15-30 mins
• Oxygen 40-60% • Prednisolone 40-50mg po od or Hydrocortisone 100mg iv qds • Nebulised β$_2$-agonist 4-6 hourly	• Continue O$_2$ and Steroids • Nebulised β$_2$-agonist with increased frequency o Salbutamol 5mg every 15-30 mins or continuous 10mg/hour • Continue ipratropium bromide nebulised 4-6 hourly until improving

STILL NOT IMPROVING

• Discuss with senior clinician and ICU
• IV Magnesium Sulphate (as above if not already given)
• Consideration by senior physician
  o iv β$_2$-agonist
  o iv aminophylline
  o IPPV

MONITORING FOR __ALL__ PATIENTS

• Repeat PEF 15-30 mins after commencing therapy
• Oximetry- maintain SpO$_2$>92%
  • Rpt ABG< 2 hours after initiation of treatment if:
    o Initial pO$_2$<8 unless subsequent S pO$_2$ >92%
    o pCO$_2$ normal/raised
    o Patient deteriorating
• Chart PEF pre- and post β$_2$-agonist and at least qds throughout hospital stay

Transfer to ICU by Doctor prepared to intubate if:
• ↓PEF
• ↓pO$_2$ or persisting hypoxia
• ↑pCO$_2$
• Exhaustion/feeble respiratory effort/confusion/drowsy
• Coma/Respiratory Arrest

Abbreviations: po- orally; iv- intravenously; PT- pneumothorax; mins- minutes; hr- hour; od- once daily; qds- six-hourly, ICU- intensive care unit; IPPV- Invasive Positive Pressure Ventilation; PEF- peak expiratory flow rate; pO$_2$- arterial partial pressure of oxygen; pCO$_2$- arterial partial pressure of Carbon Dioxide;

FIGURE 2.3. Initial management of acute severe asthma in adults in hospital. (Adapted from Annex 4 of the BTS/SIGN Asthma Guidelines).

β$_2$-Agonists

The best method of administration of β$_2$-agonists (salbutamol or albuterol in North America and terbutaline) is contentious. Use of a metered dose inhaler and spacer was as effective as nebulisation in acute severe asthma with fewer side effects.[20,21]

TABLE 2.3. Drugs recommended in the treatment of acute severe asthma, routes of administration and dosage

Medication	Route and dose
Salbutamol	**Nebulised:** 2.5–5 mg in 2.5 mL normal saline every 15–20 min until clinical improvement or continuous nebulisation at 10 mg/h (both via oxygen driven nebulisers)
	IV: 3–20 mcg/kg/h
Ipratropium bromide	**Nebulised:** 500 mcg every 6 h
Corticosteroids	**Enteral:** Prednisolone 40–60 mg once daily
	IV: Hydrocortisone 100 mg every 6 h
Aminophylline	**IV:** 5 mg/kg loading dose over 20 min (unless taking oral theophyllines) followed by 0.5–0.7 mg/kg/h infusion (guided by theophylline levels)
Magnesium sulphate	**IV:** 1.2–2 g over 20 min, one dose

Abbreviation: IV, intravenous.

However, in the most severe cases inhaler devices may be difficult to use effectively. The BTS recommends considering continuous nebulisation in severe exacerbations in which there is a poor response to nebulised β_2-agonists,[15] despite a lack of evidence of benefit in airflow obstruction, hospital admission or response.[22,23] Similarly, no difference in effectiveness has been demonstrated between the intravenous (IV) and nebulised routes, but an increase in side effects was associated with IV administration.[24]

The α-agonist action of adrenaline leading to vasoconstriction and potentially reduced airway oedema, in addition to its β-agonist action, theoretically makes it an attractive treatment option. However, comparing nebulised β_2-agonists and adrenaline demonstrated equivalent relief of airflow limitation, although the reduction in respiratory rate was greater in the β_2-agonist group.[25,26] There was no difference in side effects between the two groups and no benefit in combining the two treatments. With no proven benefit over β_2-agonists the routine use of adrenaline is not recommended.

Ipratropium Bromide

Ipratropium bromide is an anticholinergic bronchodilator with a maximum effect 60–90 min after nebulisation. Meta-analysis and a recent trial support the use of ipratropium bromide as an adjunct to

β_2-agonists in acute asthma with a larger benefit in those with severe or life-threatening asthma.[27]

Corticosteroids

Enteral steroids are as effective as parenteral and may be used providing there are no concerns regarding absorption. There is no benefit in using higher doses.[28,29]

Magnesium

A meta-analysis and systematic review assessing the benefit of intravenous magnesium sulphate in acute asthma showed no harm, but no benefit in airflow obstruction and hospital admission.[30,31] In a subgroup of patients with the most severe asthma a benefit in PEFR was observed.[30] The BTS guidelines therefore recommend giving a single dose of magnesium sulphate in patients with life-threatening asthma or in those who do not have a good initial response to inhaled brochodilators.[15]

Aminophylline

There are no data supporting the use of intravenous aminophylline as an adjunct to inhaled β_2 agonists, but side effects include palpitations, arrhythmias and vomiting.[32]

Heliox

This helium–oxygen mixture (80:20 or 70:30) has a similar viscosity to air, but a lower density. In theory this lowers resistance to flow and improves laminar flow in the airways, decreasing the work of breathing and improving the delivery of inhaled medications at a cost of decreasing the inspired oxygen concentration. Despite positive results in small studies, systematic reviews provided no evidence to support its use currently in life-threatening asthma.[15,33,34]

Leukotriene Receptor Antagonists

Oral preparations are recommended as adjuncts in the management of chronic asthma.[15] One randomised trial comparing intravenous montelukast to placebo in 194 patients with moderate to severe asthma exacerbations already receiving β_2-agonist therapy, showed improvement in FEV_1 at 10 min and 2 h.[15] Further studies are needed to confirm any benefit over standard management.

Ventilatory Support

Tracheal Intubation

If, despite maximal medical therapy, patients with severe asthma deteriorate or become exhausted, then tracheal intubation and mechanical ventilation should not be delayed even if hypercapnia is not present.[15,36] A deteriorating conscious level and impending or actual cardiopulmonary arrest are absolute indications for tracheal intubation.[15,36] Tracheal intubation rates for asthma admissions vary from 2% to 61%.[37] The process should be semi-elective and performed by an experienced team in an appropriate environment with good preparation and anticipation of the potential complications.[36] Induction of anaesthesia and positive pressure ventilation tend to further compromise venous return in asthmatic patients and may precipitate cardiovascular collapse (Figure 2.1). Fluid resuscitation and correction of electrolytes would ideally have been carried out previously. Vasoconstrictors (such as metaraminol) and the means of maintaining sedation and paralysis must be immediately available.

Anaesthetic Agents and Sedatives

Opiates may also cause dose-dependent histamine release and bronchoconstriction; fentanyl is less likely than morphine to cause histamine release. Ketamine is a general anaesthetic with sedative, analgesic and brochodilating properties, which has been used to induce anaesthesia in the emergency intubation of patients with asthma.[38] A randomised controlled trail compared the addition of ketamine or placebo in 53 patients receiving standard care in casualty. In awake patients the dose of ketamine that was tolerable in terms of the dysphoria caused, produced no bronchodilatation.[39]

Inhaled anaesthetic agents have a direct relaxant effect on bronchial smooth muscle causing bronchodilation.[40] Hypotension and myocardial irritability are the side effects of these agents, but these are minimal with sevoflurane. Numerous practical problems preclude the use of these agents in all but the most difficult cases: incompatibility with ICU ventilators, the cost of the agents and continuous anaesthetic supervision, the inability of anaesthetic ventilators to support pressures required to ventilate asthmatic patients

and finally the requirement for scavenging of the anaesthetic gases.

Neuromuscular Blocking Agents

Continued paralysis may be required to facilitate mechanical ventilation. The use of these agents is associated with an increased incidence of myopathy which appears to be exacerbated by the synergistic adverse effect of corticosteroids in patients with asthma.[41]

Mechanical Ventilation

Using a slow respiratory rate and prolonged expiratory time attenuates dynamic hyperinflation, intrinsic PEEP and the risk of air leaks (Figure 2.2). This strategy may lead to hypercapnia but this is well tolerated.[42,43] A low level of ventilator set PEEP (2/3 of PEEPi is often used) may reduce the work of breathing by improving expiratory flow. Higher levels of extrinsic PEEP may be harmful [44] and it is advisable to assess the volume of trapped gas (a facility available on some modern ventilators) associated with changes in ventilatory settings. One study of 51 patients mechanically ventilated for acute severe asthma correlated end-expiratory lung volume alone as a risk factor for the acute complications of hypotension (20%), air leaks (14%) and arrhythmias (10%).[45] In mechanically ventilated patients with uncontrolled gas trapping, manual compression of the chest wall during expiration may augment expiratory flow and lung emptying.[46,47] A less dramatic alternative is to preoxygenate the patient and then disconnect them from the inspiratory limb of the ventilator until expiratory flow ceases.

Non-invasive ventilation (NIV) has been used in small observational studies in patients with acute severe asthma with claims that physiology is improved and the outcome is unaffected.[48,49] NIV should not be used in those who are unable to cooperate and coordinate with the ventilator, those who have excessive secretions and in those in whom immediate endotracheal intubation is preferable.[36] The role of NIV is acute severe asthma is undetermined and its use cannot be recommended.

Mucous plugging and segmental or lobar collapse are common findings in asthmatic patients and the use of mucolytics and chest physiotherapy are theoretically attractive. Case reports have described the successful use of bronchoscopic lavage in refractory asthma.[50,51] There is however, significant risk associated with this procedure. Recombinant human deoxyribonuclease (a mucolytic) has been beneficial in children with refractory asthma.[52] Generous humidification should be provided to all asthmatic patients as a means to aiding expectoration.

In cases where mechanical ventilation fails to provide adequate respiratory support or is associated with uncontrollable adverse effects extracorporeal membrane oxygenation should be considered. Its successful use has been described in case reports and in the absence of right ventricular failure a veno-venous circuit should suffice.[53,54]

Discharge

In one study 16 out of 89 patients admitted to an urban ICU suffering from asthma had two or more admissions in a 3-year period.[37] Patients who have survived life-threatening asthma should receive education regarding their disease, including a written management plan. These measures reduce morbidity post-exacerbation and reduce relapse rates.[55] Regular anti-inflammatory medication should be prescribed and follow-up arranged by a respiratory specialist.[15] Table 2.4 summarises the BTS/SIGN asthma guidelines for discharge of patients admitted for acute severe asthma (Boxes 2.1 and 2.2).

TABLE 2.4. Guidelines for discharge of patients admitted with acute severe asthma

Discharge guidelines
When discharged from hospital patients should have:
• Been on inhaler medication for 24 h and have inhaler technique checked and recorded
• PEF > 75% of best/predicted and PEF diurnal variability < 25% unless discharge is agreed by a respiratory physician
• Treatment with **oral and inhaled steroids** in addition to bronchodilators
• Own PEF metre and **written asthma action plan**
• GP follow-up arranged within two working days
• Follow-up appointment in respiratory clinic within 4 weeks
Patients with severe asthma (i.e. those with need for admission) and adverse behavioural or psychosocial features are at risk of further severe or fatal attacks.
Therefore:
• Determine reason(s) for admission
• Send details of admission, discharge and potential best PEF to GP

Abbreviations: PEF, peak expiratory flow; GP, general practitioner.
Source: Adapted from BTS/SIGN Asthma Guidelines.

Box 1 Suggested further readings

- British Thoracic Society and Scottish Intercollegiate Guidelines Network. British Guideline on the Management of Asthma—A National Clinical Guideline (2008) Thorax 63 (Suppl IV): i1–107
- Rodrigo GJ, Rodrigo C, Hall JB (2004) Acute asthma in adults. A review. Chest 125(3):1081–102
- McFadden ER (2003) State of the art. Acute severe asthma. Am J Respir Crit Care Med 168:740–59

Box 2 Strategies in acute severe asthma

- Recognition of severity of asthma exacerbation and at risk groups
- Early and aggressive therapy, including adequate doses of corticosteroids
- Continued close monitoring in an appropriate setting of patients with severe exacerbations to ensure continuing response to therapy
- Avoid delays in intubation and mechanical ventilation in patients with acute severe asthma deteriorating despite maximal medical therapy
- Semi-elective intubation by experienced team in appropriate setting with anticipation of complications, especially haemodynamic compromise
- Appropriate ventilatory settings to prevent complications of mechanical ventilation
- Appropriate discharge medication, education and follow-up to prevent future exacerbations

References

1. BTS, SIGN. British Guideline on the Management of Asthma. *Thorax*. 2008 May;63 Suppl 4:iv1–121.
2. McFadden ER, Jr., Warren EL. Observations on asthma mortality. *Ann Intern Med*. 1997 Jul 15;127(2):142–7.
3. ECRHS. Variations in the prevalence of respiratory symptoms, self-reported asthma attacks, and use of asthma medication in the European Community Respiratory Health Survey (ECRHS). *Eur Respir J*. 1996 Apr;9(4):687–95.
4. Holgate S. Mediator and cytokine mechanisms in asthma. *Thorax*. 1993 Feb;48(2):103–9.
5. Larche M, Robinson DS, Kay AB. The role of T lymphocytes in the pathogenesis of asthma. *J Allergy Clin Immunol*. 2003 Mar;111(3):450–63; quiz 64.
6. Woodruff PG, Emond SD, Singh AK, Camargo CA, Jr. Sudden-onset severe acute asthma: clinical features and response to therapy. *Acad Emerg Med*. 1998 Jul;5(7):695–701.
7. Kolbe J, Fergusson W, Garrett J. Rapid onset asthma: a severe but uncommon manifestation. *Thorax*. 1998 Apr;53(4):241–7.
8. Barr RG, Woodruff PG, Clark S, Camargo CA, Jr. Sudden-onset asthma exacerbations: clinical features, response to therapy, and 2-week follow-up.

Multicenter Airway Research Collaboration (MARC) investigators. *Eur Respir J*. 2000 Feb;15(2):266–73.

9. Rodrigo GJ, Rodrigo C. Rapid-onset asthma attack: a prospective cohort study about characteristics and response to emergency department treatment. *Chest*. 2000 Dec;118(6):1547–52.

10. Marquette CH, Saulnier F, Leroy O, Wallaert B, Chopin C, Demarcq JM, et al. Long-term prognosis of near-fatal asthma. A 6-year follow-up study of 145 asthmatic patients who underwent mechanical ventilation for a near-fatal attack of asthma. *Am Rev Respir Dis*. 1992 Jul;146(1):76–81.

11. Turner MO, Noertjojo K, Vedal S, Bai T, Crump S, Fitzgerald JM. Risk factors for near-fatal asthma. A case-control study in hospitalized patients with asthma. *Am J Respir Crit Care Med*. 1998 Jun;157 (6 Pt 1):1804–9.

12. Kolbe J, Fergusson W, Vamos M, Garrett J. Case-control study of severe life threatening asthma (SLTA) in adults: demographics, health care, and management of the acute attack. *Thorax*. 2000 Dec;55(12): 1007–15.

13. Sur S, Crotty TB, Kephart GM, Hyma BA, Colby TV, Reed CE, et al. Sudden-onset fatal asthma. A distinct entity with few eosinophils and relatively more neutrophils in the airway submucosa? *Am Rev Respir Dis*. 1993 Sep;148(3):713–9.

14. Wasserfallen JB, Schaller MD, Feihl F, Perret CH. Sudden asphyxic asthma: a distinct entity? *Am Rev Respir Dis*. 1990 Jul;142(1):108–11.

15. Reid LM. The presence or absence of bronchial mucus in fatal asthma. *J Allergy Clin Immunol*. 1987 Sep;80(3 Pt 2):415–6.

16. Papiris S, Kotanidou A, Malagari K, Roussos C. Clinical review: severe asthma. *Crit Care*. 2002 Feb;6(1):30–44.

17. Rodriguez-Roisin R. Acute severe asthma: pathophysiology and pathobiology of gas exchange abnormalities. *Eur Respir J*. 1997 Jun;10(6):1359–71.

18. Corbridge TC, Hall JB. The assessment and management of adults with status asthmaticus. *Am J Respir Crit Care Med*. 1995 May;151(5):1296–316.

19. Wareham NJ, Harrison BD, Jenkins PF, Nicholls J, Stableforth DE. A district confidential enquiry into deaths due to asthma. *Thorax*. 1993 Nov;48(11): 1117–20.

20. Kolbe J, Vamos M, Fergusson W, Elkind G. Determinants of management errors in acute severe asthma. *Thorax*. 1998 Jan;53(1):14–20.

21. Anderson HR, Ayres JG, Sturdy PM, Bland JM, Butland BK, Peckitt C, et al. Bronchodilator treatment and deaths from asthma: case-control study. *Bmj*. 2005 Jan 15;330(7483):117.

22. Innes NJ, Reid A, Halstead J, Watkin SW, Harrison BD. Psychosocial risk factors in near-fatal asthma

and in asthma deaths. *J R Coll Physicians Lond*. 1998 Sep-Oct;32(5):430–4.

23. Plaza V, Serrano J, Picado C, Sanchis J. Frequency and clinical characteristics of rapid-onset fatal and near-fatal asthma. *Eur Respir J*. 2002 May;19(5):846–52.

24. Kallenbach JM, Frankel AH, Lapinsky SE, Thornton AS, Blott JA, Smith C, et al. Determinants of near fatality in acute severe asthma. *Am J Med*. 1993 Sep;95(3):265–72.

25. Richards GN, Kolbe J, Fenwick J, Rea HH. Demographic characteristics of patients with severe life threatening asthma: comparison with asthma deaths. *Thorax*. 1993 Nov;48(11):1105–9.

26. White CS, Cole RP, Lubetsky HW, Austin JH. Acute asthma. Admission chest radiography in hospitalized adult patients. *Chest*. 1991 Jul;100(1):14–6.

27. Rodrigo C, Rodrigo G. Salbutamol treatment of acute severe asthma in the ED: MDI versus hand-held nebulizer. *Am J Emerg Med*. 1998 Nov;16(7):637–42.

28. Raimondi AC, Schottlender J, Lombardi D, Molfino NA. Treatment of acute severe asthma with inhaled albuterol delivered via jet nebulizer, metered dose inhaler with spacer, or dry powder. *Chest*. 1997 Jul;112(1):24–8.

29. Rodrigo GJ, Rodrigo C. Continuous vs intermittent beta-agonists in the treatment of acute adult asthma: a systematic review with meta-analysis. *Chest*. 2002 Jul;122(1):160–5.

30. Papo MC, Frank J, Thompson AE. A prospective, randomized study of continuous versus intermittent nebulized albuterol for severe status asthmaticus in children. *Crit Care Med*. 1993 Oct;21(10):1479–86.

31. Wang DL, Tang CC, Wung BS, Chen HH, Hung MS, Wang JJ. Cyclical strain increases endothelin-1 secretion and gene expression in human endothelial cells. *Biochem Biophys Res Commun*. 1993 Sep 15;195(2):1050–6.

32. Rudnitsky GS, Eberlein RS, Schoffstall JM, Mazur JE, Spivey WH. Comparison of intermittent and continuously nebulized albuterol for treatment of asthma in an urban emergency department. *Ann Emerg Med*. 1993 Dec;22(12):1842–6.

33. Innes NJ, Stocking JA, Daynes TJ, Harrison BD. Randomised pragmatic comparison of UK and US treatment of acute asthma presenting to hospital. *Thorax*. 2002 Dec;57(12):1040–4.

34. Travers AH, Rowe BH, Barker S, Jones A, Camargo CA, Jr. The effectiveness of IV beta-agonists in treating patients with acute asthma in the emergency department: a meta-analysis. *Chest*. 2002 Oct;122(4): 1200–7.

35. Abroug F, Nouira S, Bchir A, Boujdaria R, Elatrous S, Bouchoucha S. A controlled trial of nebulized salbutamol and adrenaline in acute severe asthma. *Intensive Care Med*. 1995 Jan;21(1):18–23.

36. Adoun M, Frat JP, Dore P, Rouffineau J, Godet C, Robert R. Comparison of nebulized epinephrine and terbutaline in patients with acute severe asthma: a controlled trial. *J Crit Care*. 2004 Jun;19(2):99–102.

37. Rodrigo G, Rodrigo C, Burschtin O. A meta-analysis of the effects of ipratropium bromide in adults with acute asthma. *Am J Med*. 1999 Oct;107(4):363–70.

38. FitzGerald M. Acute asthma. *Bmj*. 2001 Oct 13;323 (7317):841–5.

39. Rowe BH, Spooner C, Ducharme FM, Bretzlaff JA, Bota GW. Early emergency department treatment of acute asthma with systemic corticosteroids. *Cochrane Database Syst Rev*. 2001(1):CD002178.

40. Manser R, Reid D, Abramson M. Corticosteroids for acute severe asthma in hospitalised patients. *Cochrane Database Syst Rev*. 2001(1):CD001740.

41. Rodrigo G, Rodrigo C, Burschtin O. Efficacy of magnesium sulfate in acute adult asthma: a meta-analysis of randomized trials. *Am J Emerg Med*. 2000 Mar;18(2):216–21.

42. Rowe BH, Bretzlaff JA, Bourdon C, Bota GW, Camargo CA, Jr. Magnesium sulfate for treating exacerbations of acute asthma in the emergency department. *Cochrane Database Syst Rev*. 2000(2): CD001490.

43. Alter HJ. Intravenous magnesium as an adjuvant in acute bronchospasm: A meta-analysis. *Annals of Emergency Medicine*. 2000;36(3):191–7.

44. Parameswaran K, Belda J, Rowe BH. Addition of intravenous aminophylline to beta2-agonists in adults with acute asthma. *Cochrane Database Syst Rev*. 2000(4):CD002742.

45. Rodrigo G, Pollack C, Rodrigo C, Rowe BH. Heliox for nonintubated acute asthma patients. *Cochrane Database Syst Rev*. 2003(4):CD002884.

46. Ho AM, Lee A, Karmakar MK, Dion PW, Chung DC, Contardi LH. Heliox vs air-oxygen mixtures for the treatment of patients with acute asthma: a systematic overview. *Chest*. 2003 Mar;123(3):882–90.

47. Reuben AD, Harris AR. Heliox for asthma in the emergency department: a review of the literature. *Emergency Medicine Journal*. 2004;21:131–5.

48. Camargo CA, Jr., Smithline HA, Malice MP, Green SA, Reiss TF. A randomized controlled trial of intravenous montelukast in acute asthma. *Am J Respir Crit Care Med*. 2003 Feb 15;167(4):528–33.

49. Phipps P, Garrard CS. The pulmonary physician in critical care . 12: Acute severe asthma in the intensive care unit. *Thorax*. 2003 Jan;58(1):81–8.

50. Wort SJ. The management of acute severe asthma in adults. Current Anaesthesia and Critical Care. [Review]. 2003;14(2):81–9.

51. Afessa B, Morales I, Cury JD. Clinical course and outcome of patients admitted to an ICU for status asthmaticus. *Chest*. 2001 Nov;120(5):1616–21.

52. Sarma VJ. Use of ketamine in acute severe asthma. *Acta Anaesthesiol Scand*. 1992 Jan;36(1):106–7.

53. L'Hommedieu CS, Arens JJ. The use of ketamine for the emergency intubation of patients with status asthmaticus. *Ann Emerg Med*. 1987 May;16(5):568–71.

54. Howton JC, Rose J, Duffy S, Zoltanski T, Levitt MA. Randomized, double-blind, placebo-controlled trial of intravenous ketamine in acute asthma. *Ann Emerg Med*. 1996 Feb;27(2):170–5.

55. Hirshman CA, Edelstein G, Peetz S, Wayne R, Downes H. Mechanism of action of inhalational anesthesia on airways. *Anesthesiology*. 1982 Feb;56(2):107–11.

56. Korenaga S, Takeda K, Ito Y. Differential effects of halothane on airway nerves and muscle. *Anesthesiology*. 1984 Apr;60(4):309–18.

57. Behbehani NA, Al-Mane F, D'Yachkova Y, Pare P, FitzGerald JM. Myopathy following mechanical ventilation for acute severe asthma: the role of muscle relaxants and corticosteroids. *Chest*. 1999 Jun;115(6):1627–31.

58. Leatherman JW, Fluegel WL, David WS, Davies SF, Iber C. Muscle weakness in mechanically ventilated patients with severe asthma. *Am J Respir Crit Care Med*. 1996 May;153(5):1686–90.

59. Mutlu GM, Factor P, Schwartz DE, Sznajder JI. Severe status asthmaticus: management with permissive hypercapnia and inhalation anesthesia. *Crit Care Med*. 2002 Feb;30(2):477–80.

60. Feihl F, Perret C. Permissive hypercapnia. How permissive should we be? *Am J Respir Crit Care Med*. 1994 Dec;150(6 Pt 1):1722–37.

61. Tuxen DV. Detrimental effects of positive end-expiratory pressure during controlled mechanical ventilation of patients with severe airflow obstruction. *Am Rev Respir Dis*. 1989 Jul;140(1):5–9.

62. Williams TJ, Tuxen DV, Scheinkestel CD, Czarny D, Bowes G. Risk factors for morbidity in mechanically ventilated patients with acute severe asthma. *Am Rev Respir Dis*. 1992 Sep;146(3):607–15.

63. Fisher MM, Bowey CJ, Ladd-Hudson K. External chest compression in acute asthma: a preliminary study. *Crit Care Med*. 1989 Jul;17(7):686–7.

64. Eason J, Tayler D, Cottam S, Edwards R, Beard C, Peachey T, et al. Manual chest compression for total bronchospasm. *The Lancet*. 1991;337:366.

65. Shivaram U, Miro AM, Cash ME, Finch PJ, Heurich AE, Kamholz SL. Cardiopulmonary responses to continuous positive airway pressure in acute asthma. *J Crit Care*. 1993 Jun;8(2):87–92.

66. Meduri GU, Cook TR, Turner RE, Cohen M, Leeper KV. Noninvasive positive pressure ventilation in status asthmaticus. *Chest*. 1996 Sep;110(3):767–74.

67. Soroksky A, Stav D, Shpirer I. A pilot prospective, randomized, placebo-controlled trial of bilevel

positive airway pressure in acute asthmatic attack. *Chest*. 2003 Apr;123(4):1018–25.

68. Lang D, Simon R, Mathison D, Timms R, Stevenson D. Safety and possible efficacy of fiberoptic bronchoscopy with lavage in the management of refractory asthma with mucous empaction. *Annals of Allergy*. 1991;67:324–30.

69. Karnik A, Medhat M, Farah S. Therapeutic use of brochoalveolar lavage in a very difficult asthmatic: *a case report Journal of Asthma*. 1989;26(3):181–4.

70. Patel A, Harrison E, Durward A, Murdoch IA. Intratracheal recombinant human deoxyribonuclease in acute life-threatening asthma refractory to conventional treatment. *Br J Anaesth*. 2000 Apr;84(4):505–7.

71. Tajimi K, Kasai T, Nakatani T, Kobayashi K. Extracorporeal lung assist for patient with hypercapnia due to status asthmaticus. *Intensive Care Med*. 1988; 14(5):588–9.

72. Shapiro MB, Kleaveland AC, Bartlett RH. Extracorporeal life support for status asthmaticus. *Chest*. 1993 Jun;103(6):1651–4.

73. Cowie RL, Revitt SG, Underwood MF, Field SK. The effect of a peak flow-based action plan in the prevention of exacerbations of asthma. *Chest*. 1997 Dec; 112(6):1534–8.

3
Chronic Obstructive Airways Disease

Richard Leach

Abstract Chronic obstructive pulmonary disease (COPD) is a slowly progressive disease characterised by increasing cough, wheeze and exertional breathlessness with associated airflow obstruction that is not fully reversible. The majority of patients have a 20-pack-year history of cigarette smoking. Typically, progressive decline in lung function with intermittent acute exacerbations leads to chronic respiratory symptoms, disability and respiratory failure. The term COPD encompasses varying combinations of pulmonary emphysema, chronic bronchitis and chronic severe asthma, and it may be difficult to define the relative importance of each in an individual patient. Over the last 10 years there have been numerous COPD guidelines published, many of which differ in detail. This chapter includes guidelines from the National Institute for Clinical Excellence (NICE, UK)[1], the ATS/ERS standards for the diagnosis and treatment of patients with COPD position paper[2], the National Institute for Health (USA) Global Initiative for Chronic Obstructive Lung Disease[3], the British Thoracic Society Guidelines[4], the American Thoracic Society guidelines[5] and a BMJ review[6].

Epidemiology

In 1999, there were 30,000 deaths attributable to chronic obstructive pulmonary disease (COPD) in the UK, representing 5.1% of all deaths (sixth commonest cause of death). A diagnosis of COPD has been established in 0.9 million of the UK population (~1.5%) most of whom are over 45 years old, although the true prevalence is probably >1.5 million (i.e. >40% of cases are unidentified). Worldwide, COPD is currently the fourth leading cause of death. It is the only preventable cause of death that is increasing. The age-adjusted death rate as a proportion of the 1965 rate is 163% (compared to a 59% reduction for ischaemic heart disease). Currently, COPD exacerbations account for ~10% of all emergency hospital medical admissions and are more frequent in the winter months. The NHS COPD budget is £818 million/year (~£800/patient/year). However, total economic costs for the UK are over £2 billion/year when lost working days and social service support budgets are included. *Prognosis*: yearly mortality is ~25% when FEV_1 is <0.8 L. This is increased by coexisting cor pulmonale, hypercapnea and weight loss.

Definitions

COPD is a preventable and treatable disease state characterised by airflow limitation that is not fully reversible. The airflow limitation is usually both progressive and associated with an abnormal inflammatory response of the lungs to noxious particles or gases, primarily caused by cigarette smoking. Although COPD affects the lungs, it also produces significant systemic consequences (ATS/ERS). *Chronic bronchitis* is 'the presence of chronic cough and sputum production for at least 3 months of 2 consecutive years in the absence of other diseases recognised to cause sputum production'. This definition was used by the MRC as an epidemiological definition of 'chronic bronchitis'. However, it does not always signify the presence of airways obstruction or the diagnosis of COPD. Most of the morbidities and mortalities of COPD relate to airways obstruction and not mucus hypersecretion.

Pathogenesis

Smoking and other risk factors accelerate normal age-related decline in expiratory airflow (Table 3.1). *Deficiency of α_1-antitrypsin* is associated with early onset emphysema and occurs in 2% of COPD patients. α_1-Antitrypsin is a protease inhibitor which prevents alveolar damage. Normal α_1-antitrypsin production occurs in subjects with two M genes (i.e. phenotype MM). However, several genes including Z and S cause α_1-antitrypsin deficiency. Homozygotes (e.g. ZZ, SS) have very low plasma α_1-antitrypsin levels and may develop emphysema in the third or fourth decade of life, whereas heterozygotes (e.g. MS, MZ) have reduced levels and may be at greater risk of emphysema, particularly in smokers.

Pathophysiology

Although emphysema and chronic bronchitis often coexist they are different disease processes.

- *Emphysema* is associated with destruction of alveolar septa and capillaries and may be due to inadequate anti-protease defences against inhaled toxins (e.g. tobacco smoke). Smoking causes centrilobular emphysema with predominantly upper lobe involvement, whereas α_1-antitrypsin deficiency causes panacinar emphysema, which affects the lower lobes. Loss of lung tissue creates bullae (large airspaces), reduces lung elastic recoil and impairs diffusion

TABLE 3.1. Risk factors for COPD

- Smoking
- Age > 50 years: prevalence ~5–10%
- Male gender
- Childhood chest infections
- Airway hyperreactivity—asthma/atopy
- Low socio-economic status
- α_1-Anti-trypsin deficiency
- Heavy metal exposure—cadmium
- Atmospheric pollution

capacity. Emphysematous airways obstruction is caused by distal airways collapse during expiration due to loss of the 'elastic' radial traction from the surrounding lung tissue that normally maintains airway patency (Figure 3.1a)[7]. *'Static' hyperinflation* describes the alveolar air trapping that occurs under resting conditions due to this distal airways collapse (Figures 3.1a and 3.2). *'Dynamic' hyperinflation* describes the additional air trapping that occurs when bronchoconstriction (e.g. asthma, COPD exacerbations), exercise or rapid ventilation (either spontaneous or mechanical ventilation [MV]) reduce expiratory (± inspiratory) times and further impair alveolar emptying (Figures 3.2a and b). Hyperinflation increases 'end-expiratory alveolar pressure' (auto-PEEP, see below) enhancing expiratory airflow but the 'horizontal' position of the ribs and the flat diaphragm place the inspiratory musculature at a mechanical disadvantage, which increases the elastic work of breathing. Raised intrathoracic pressure associated with hyperinflation reduces venous return to the heart and cardiac output leading to cardiovascular instability.

- *Auto-PEEP* (Figure 3.3) refers to the component of positive end-expiratory pressure (PEEP) during mechanical ventilation that is due to 'dynamic' hyperinflation and represents the pressure of the trapped alveolar gas. The pressure applied to the airway by the clinician is called PEEP (sometimes called 'extrinsic' PEEP). The pressure measured when all airflows are stopped at end expiration is equivalent to the average alveolar pressure and is termed the 'total' PEEP. Auto-PEEP is the difference between the 'total' PEEP and PEEP (i.e. that component of 'total' PEEP attributable to dynamic hyperinflation). Confusingly, the term 'intrinsic' PEEP may be used to refer to auto-PEEP or 'total' PEEP. 'Total' PEEP and thus auto-PEEP is usually measured by occluding the expiratory port of the ventilator at end expiration for ~2 s. There is probably considerable regional variation in auto-PEEP and the measured end-expiratory value is the mean (Figure 3.3). Auto-PEEP measured at end expiration may also be misleadingly low, as it reflects only those pressures in alveoli that communicate with the airway (Figure 3.3). The end-inspiratory plateau pressure

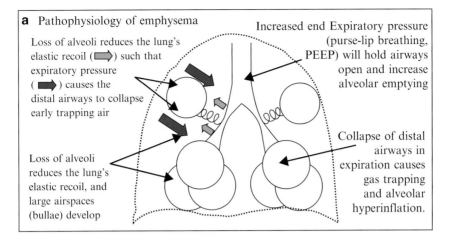

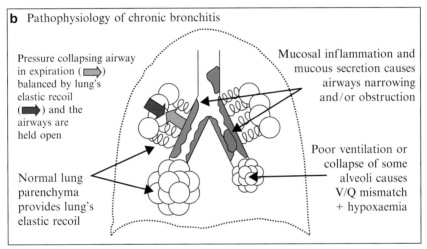

FIGURE 3.1. Pathophysiology of emphysema and chronic bronchitis.

is usually uniform (i.e. there is little regional variation) and may be a better indicator of gas trapping (e.g. at different respiratory rates) when tidal volume and PEEP are fixed. A high plateau pressure despite a normal or low tidal volume indicates widespread gas trapping. A marked disparity between a high plateau pressure and a low auto-PEEP measured by end-expiratory occlusion suggests extensive airways obstruction due to inflammation or mucus plugging (Figure 3.3).

- *Chronic bronchitis* causes airways obstruction due to chronic mucosal inflammation (± airways damage), mucus gland hypertrophy with mucus hypersecretion and bronchospasm (Figure 3.1b). The lung parenchyma is unaffected. V/Q mismatch occurs due to poor ventilation of alveoli due to early airways closure in expiration or due to alveolar collapse if the airway is completely obstructed (Figures 3.1b, 3.2a and b).

Diagnosis

Diagnosis should be considered in any patient who has symptoms of cough, wheeze, sputum production (or 'winter bronchitis'), exertional dyspnoea and/or a history of risk factors (e.g. smoking, occupation). Weight loss, ankle oedema, nocturnal waking and fatigue should be assessed. Haemoptysis or chest pain is infrequent in COPD and raises the

a

Time constant (TC) determines alveolar filling

Time constant = compliance x resistance

- Non compliant alveoli have short TC
- Alveoli with narrowed airways have long TC

A short inspiratory time: results in incomplete inflation of alveoli with narrowed airways causing V/Q mismatching and hypoxaemia

Non-compliant alveolus

Normal alveolus

Volume

Alveolus with airways narrowing

Inpiration   **Expiration**

b

A long expiratory time is required to prevent gas trapping because the rate of alveolar deflation in decreased due to:

1. Airways obstruction: which slows expiration. A short expiratory time causes incomplete alveolar emptying (gas trapping).

Reduced Airflow

10

2. Distal airways collapse: initially reduces airflow and then causes gas trapping (Fig 2)

10

↑pressure here (PEEP) will hold the airways open allowing ↑alveolar emptying

The pressure of the trapped gas (auto-PEEP) can be measured at end expiration by occluding the expiratory limb of the ventilator

A reduction in breath rate (8-10/min) increases both inspiratory and expiratory times

c

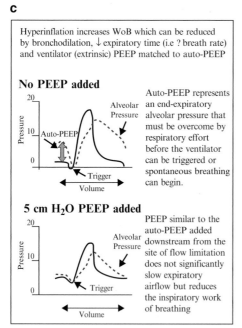

Hyperinflation increases WoB which can be reduced by bronchodilation, ↓ expiratory time (i.e ? breath rate) and ventilator (extrinsic) PEEP matched to auto-PEEP

No PEEP added

Pressure

20

10

Auto-PEEP

0

Trigger

Volume

Alveolar Pressure

Auto-PEEP represents an end-expiratory alveolar pressure that must be overcome by respiratory effort before the ventilator can be triggered or spontaneous breathing can begin.

5 cm H$_2$O PEEP added

Pressure

20

10

0

Trigger

Volume

Alveolar Pressure

PEEP similar to the auto-PEEP added downstream from the site of flow limitation does not significantly slow expiratory airflow but reduces the inspiratory work of breathing

FIGURE 3.2. Pathophysiology and strategies during mechanical ventilation to a) improve alvedar filling, b) aid alveolar deflation and c) correct for hyperinflation and auto-PEEP.

possibility of alternative diagnoses. The diagnosis is confirmed by spirometry, which demonstrates a post-bronchodilator FEV$_1$ < 80% of the predicted value in combination with airflow obstruction (FEV$_1$/FVC ratio < 0.7) that is largely irreversible with bronchodilator therapy or following steroid

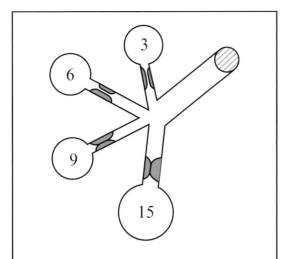

There is considerable variation in auto-PEEP. The greatest tendency for airways closure and air trapping occurs in the dependent regions.

Although end-expiratory airways occlusion reflects the average auto-PEEP among open alveolar units (i.e. in this example 3,6,9 = average 6), the highest levels of auto-PEEP are found in alveoli cutoff from the airway (i.e. in this example 15)

FIGURE 3.3.   Auto-PEEP.

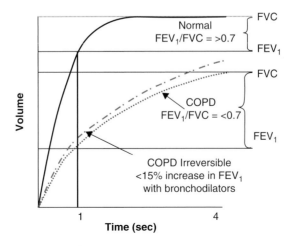

FIGURE 3.4.   Spirometry in normal and COPD patients illustrating that airflow obstruction is irreversible with bronchodilators ($\pm$ steroids) in COPD.

therapy (i.e. <15% increase in FEV_1) (Figure 3.4). The severity of COPD is classified by (a) FEV_1 as a percentage of predicted (e.g. BTS guidelines: mild 50–80%; moderate 30–49%; severe <30% predicted; but individual classifications differ); and (b) by severity of symptoms (e.g. at risk; intermittent or persistent symptoms; frequent exacerbations; respiratory failure). Routine assessment includes blood tests and chest radiograph. The clinical scenario determines the need for further investigation (e.g. α_1-antitrypsin, gas transfer, lung volumes, CT scan, sputum culture, ECG).

- *Emphysema*: this is associated with normal resting blood gases because alveolar septa and capillaries are destroyed in proportion to each other. Desaturation during exercise and increased minute ventilation are due to reduced diffusion capacity. Lung function tests confirm impaired diffusion (D_{LCO}, K_{CO}) and increased lung volumes (TLC, FRC, RV). Chest radiography (CXR) reveals hyperinflation (e.g. flat diaphragms, large retrosternal airspace), narrow mediastinum, bullae, hyperlucency and reduced peripheral vascular markings. Patients with emphysema are often relatively well oxygenated, but breathless and cachexic with hyperinflated chests and are classically described as 'pink-puffers'.
- *Chronic bronchitis*: the diffusion capacity and lung volumes are usually normal but V/Q mismatch due to poor alveolar ventilation or collapse may cause hypoxaemia with associated pulmonary hypertension (PHT) and fluid retention. CXR shows increased vascular markings but normal lung volumes. Because these patients are often hypoxaemic and oedematous but not breathless, they are sometimes described as 'blue-bloaters'. In reality, most patients with COPD have varying degrees of emphysema and bronchitis and a mixed clinical picture (see below).

Clinical Features

The concept of emphysematous 'pink-puffers' and bronchitic 'blue-bloaters' is unreliable as most patients have coexistent elements of both disease processes and a mixed clinical picture (i.e. 'blue-puffers'). Emphysematous patients tend to be breathless and tachypnoic, with signs of hyperinflation and

malnutrition including thin body, barrel chest, pursed-lip breathing and accessory muscle use. Chest auscultation reveals distant breath sounds and prolonged expiratory wheeze. Chronic bronchitic patients are often less breathless despite potential hypoxaemia, and reduced respiratory drive leads to CO_2 retention with associated bounding pulse, vasodilation, confusion, headache, flapping tremor and papilloedema. Hypoxaemia-induced renal fluid retention, rather than right heart failure, is the cause of oedema and the clinical picture of 'cor pulmonale' (i.e. hepatomegaly, ankle oedema, raised CVP). Pulmonary hypertension (PHT) is a late feature. It occurs earlier in bronchitic patients due to hypoxic pulmonary vasoconstriction and is partially reversed by oxygen therapy. In emphysema, extensive capillary loss may contribute to PHT.

General Management

Recent guidelines [1–4] and UK national priorities for healthcare require (a) *early diagnosis*: by establishing smoking history and monitoring spirometry (± reversibility) in >90% of primary care populations (see above); (b) *prevention of disease progression*: by encouraging smoking cessation and reducing other risk factors (e.g. occupational dust exposure, environmental pollution); (c) *optimisation of medical therapy*: to improve quality and length of life in stable COPD and to prevent acute exacerbations and associated hospital admissions;[7,8,9] and (d) *early hospital discharge*: with ongoing community support (e.g. COPD outreach teams).

Management of Stable COPD

The exact sequence of initiation of available therapies differs slightly between individual guidelines (e.g. GOLD, BTS, NICE) but Figure 3.5 provides a clinically useful synthesis of the different management protocols for stable COPD (adapted from [6]).

Non-pharmacological Therapy

- *Smoking cessation* is the single, most effective (and cost-effective) intervention to reduce the

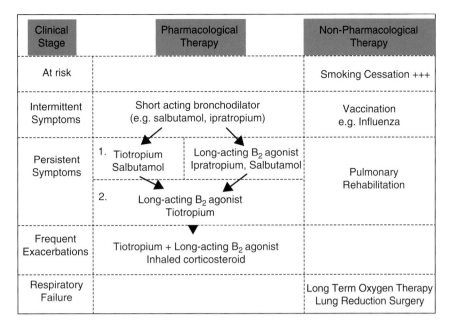

FIGURE 3.5. Clinical algorithm for COPD management.

risk of developing COPD and to stop its progression. Even a 3-min period of counselling urging a smoker to 'quit' in a clear, strong and personalised manner can be effective, and at the very least this should be done for every smoker at every visit. Further success is reported with support schemes (e.g. ASH, NHS) and anti-smoking pharmacotherapy (e.g. nicotine replacement therapy, bupropion).

- *Pulmonary rehabilitation* strengthens respiratory muscles, increases exercise tolerance, reduces hospitalisations, enhances quality of life, increases physical and emotional participation in everyday activities and reduces symptoms. These benefits are achieved by improving education (e.g. breathing techniques), addressing altered mood and social isolation and preventing weight loss, muscle wasting and exercise deconditioning. For example, during an acute, non-infective exacerbation of COPD a patient may be taught how to partially relieve dyspnoea by (a) splinting the shoulder girdle to assist work of breathing and (b) slowing respiratory rate to allow longer expiration with combined 'pursed-lip' breathing to 'splint' open small airways during expiration thus reducing air trapping and allowing larger subsequent inspiratory volumes.

- *Nutrition* is related to body mass index (BMI), which should be monitored and maintained in the range >20 to <25. When BMI is <20, improving nutritional status improves respiratory muscle strength and prognosis. Similarly, when BMI is >25, reducing weight improves functional status and reduces dyspnoea.

Pharmacological Therapy

- *Bronchodilators* (Figure 3.5) are central to the symptomatic management of COPD[7,8,9]. Initially prescribed on an as required basis to relieve symptoms, they are subsequently given regularly to prevent or relieve symptoms. When given by the preferred inhaled route, attention to inhaler technique is essential and side effects are mild, predictable and dose-dependent. Although spirometric improvements with inhaled bronchodilators are small, recent studies show reductions in functional residual capacity (FRC) and hyperinflation, which correlate with improved functional status, dyspnoea index and quality-of-life measures. *Nebuliser therapy*: patients with distressing breathlessness despite maximal inhaler therapy should be considered for home nebuliser therapy with regular review.

(a) *Inhaled β₂-agonists* have a rapid onset of action (<5 min) and are initially prescribed as short-acting, cheaper agents (e.g. salbutamol, albuterol). As COPD severity progresses regular long-acting agents (e.g. salmeterol, e-fomoterol) may be more convenient and have been demonstrated to improve health status.

(b) *Inhaled anticholinergics agents* have a slower onset of action (maximum effect ~60 min) than β₂-agonists, but are equally effective (or better) bronchodilators in COPD. Both short-acting (e.g. ipratropium bromide) and long-acting (e.g. tiotropium bromide) anticholinergic agents improve health status and reduce hyperinflation. Tiotropium bromide, a once daily therapy, is superior to ipratropium bromide as it acts specifically on the M3 bronchodilator muscurinic receptor, whereas ipratropium bromide acts on three muscurinic receptors M1, M2 and M3, where M1 and M3 receptors are bronchodilators and M2 is bronchoconstrictor[8]. Recent studies have confirmed that tiotropium is more effective than ipratropium and may have benefits compared to long-acting β₂-agonists. Combinations of β₂-agonists and anticholinergic agents are additive with greater effect than either agent alone and fewer side effects.

(c) *Methylxanthines* (e.g. theophylline, aminophylline) are usually prescribed as slow-release oral preparations and improve exercise tolerance and blood gases but have negligible effects on spirometry. In addition to their bronchodilator effects they may improve respiratory drive, diaphragmatic strength and mucociliary clearance. However, due to potential toxicity and the need for monitoring of plasma levels at higher doses, inhaled bronchodilators are preferred when available.

- *Inhaled corticosteroids* do not reduce long-term decline in FEV₁ in patients with COPD. In mild and moderate COPD long-term treatment with inhaled corticosteroids is only recommended if a previous trial of inhaled or oral steroids has shown a beneficial spirometric response. However, the combination of an inhaled corticosteroid with a long-acting β₂-agonist is recommended in patients with an FEV₁ < 50% predicted

who have had two or more exacerbations requiring oral steroids (± antibiotics) over the previous 12 months, as this has been demonstrated to decrease the frequency of further exacerbations. Long-term treatment with *oral corticosteroids* is not recommended in COPD and benefits less than 25% of patients. Steroid-induced myopathy and other systemic side effects of oral steroids may contribute to muscle weakness and early respiratory failure.

- *Vaccination* against influenza and pneumococcal infection is essential. In COPD patients, influenza vaccination reduces serious illness and death due to influenza by ~50%.

- *Other pharmacological therapies include the following*:

(a) *Mucolytics* assist a few patients with excessive sputum production.

(b) *Antitussive agents* are not recommended in COPD as cough has a significant protective effect.

(c) *Conventional antidepressant pharmacotherapy* should be considered in severely depressed COPD patients.

(d) *Benzodiazepines and narcotics* are respiratory depressants and may worsen hypercapnia. They are not recommended except in end-stage, palliative COPD when they may help relieve severe dyspnoea.

(e) *α₁-Antitrypsin therapy* is expensive, of unproven value and is not recommended for routine use (NICE, BTS). Patients should be referred to specialist centres for advice.

(f) *Other therapies* such as antioxidants, respiratory stimulants, regular antibiotics and immunoregulators are not recommended in stable COPD.

Long-Term Oxygen Therapy (LTOT)

- LTOT used for >15 h/day improves survival in hypoxaemic patients. It may also have beneficial effects on haemodynamics, haematological characteristics, exercise capacity and mental state. It is only recommended when PaO₂ is <7.3 kPa with or without hypercapnia in clinically stable COPD patients. When PaO₂ is >7.3 kPa but <8 kPa, LTOT may be appropriate if one of secondary polycythaemia, nocturnal hypoxaemia, peripheral oedema or pulmonary hypertension is present. It should only be prescribed after full assessment by a respiratory physician.

Surgery

- Bullectomy is effective in reducing dyspnoea and improving lung function in carefully selected patients. Lung volume reduction surgery or transplantation may be indicated in advanced COPD, but long-term efficacy and selection criteria are not established.

Management of Acute Exacerbations

Acute exacerbations are common, and when severe may require admission to hospital (± critical care facilities). An acute exacerbation is defined as a sustained worsening of the patient's usual stable state that is acute in onset and includes worsening breathlessness, cough, increased sputum production and discoloured sputum. The cause is often unknown but infection, pulmonary embolism, pneumothorax, coexisting ischaemic heart disease, heart failure and arrhythmias (e.g. atrial fibrillation due to atrial enlargement, medications or metabolic disturbances) can precipitate exacerbations. Frequent exacerbations increase the rate of decline in FEV_1 and lung function. Average cost of a severe COPD exacerbation (usually with hospital admission) is about £1,500. Following hospital admission with an acute exacerbation, the readmission rate is >30% and mortality is >10% within 3 months. Following ICU admission 12-month mortality is ~40%.

General Measures

- *Oxygen therapy (OT)* is essential in all acute COPD exacerbations and the small increase in $PaCO_2$ that occurs in most cases is of no consequence. Unfortunately, ~10% of COPD patients Unfortunately, ~10% of COPD patients with impaired ventilatory mechanisms develop hypoventilation and CO_2 retention with OT. Nevertheless, these patients still benefit from low-dose 'controlled' OT (24–28%), as they are on the steep part of the oxy-haemoglobin dissociation curve where small increases in PaO_2

do not cause much CO_2 retention but significantly increase arterial oxygen content. In controlled OT, the response to increasing oxygen concentrations is monitored with arterial blood gas (ABG) measurements to achieve a PaO_2 > 8 kPa without a substantial rise in $PaCO_2$.

(a) *Prehospital OT:* in the absence of an oximeter or ABG measurements the initial selection of an appropriate dose of O_2 is difficult. During the short period (<20 min) of prehospital transport and A + E department assessment, continuous 40% O_2 therapy should be started and if an oximeter is available, it should be adjusted to maintain SaO_2 > 88% but <93%. Controlled OT using a fixed performance (24–28%) 'Venturi' mask may be preferable if drowsiness develops or if type 2 respiratory failure has occurred previously.

(b) *After blood gas measurement:* OT is best given via a Venturi mask and is titrated to the lowest concentration required to achieve an SaO_2 88–92% (PaO_2 ~ 8 kPa). Higher SaO_2 has no advantage but may cause or exacerbate hypercapnia and respiratory acidosis. ABG must be monitored regularly. If $PaCO_2$ rises (>8 kPa), pH falls (<7.35), or if the patient becomes drowsy or fatigued, non-invasive positive pressure ventilation (NIPPV) should be initiated (see below). If hypercapnia and respiratory acidosis progress but intubation and mechanical ventilation are considered inappropriate (i.e. end-stage disease), FiO_2 is reduced to stimulate hypoxic drive and spontaneous ventilation, thereby decreasing $PaCO_2$. SaO_2 will fall to <88% but aim to maintain PaO_2 at >6.5 kPa (SaO_2 80–85%).

- *Respiratory/physiotherapy* assists secretion clearance (e.g. breathing and coughing techniques).
- *Fluid, electrolyte and nutrition management* is especially difficult in 'cor pulmonale' and requires careful monitoring. Electrolyte correction (e.g. hypophosphataemia, hypokalaemia) and good nutrition (2,000 cal intake daily) improve respiratory muscle strength and endurance. Although it is possible to generate excessive CO_2 production by overfeeding with carbohydrate, this is rarely a problem. Low carbohydrate, high lipid

feeds (to reduce CO_2 generation) are rarely necessary. Thromboembolic prophylaxis is essential in immobile patients.

Pharmacological Therapy

- **Bronchodilators**: high-dose, aerosolised, short-acting β-agonists and anticholinergic bronchodilators, usually delivered by nebuliser, relieve symptoms and improve gas exchange. Nebulisers should be driven with compressed air in hypercapnic patients. Patients should be changed to handheld inhalers as soon as their condition has stabilised.
- **Oral corticosteroids**: in the absence of contraindications, oral corticosteroids improve lung function and hasten recovery and should be used, in conjunction with other therapies, in all patients with an exacerbation of COPD. Early therapy maximises benefit. Prednisolone 30 mg orally should be prescribed for 7–14 days. Osteoporosis prophylaxis should be considered in patients requiring frequent courses of steroids.
- **Antibiotic therapy**: meta-analysis data suggest a small morbidity and mortality advantage with antibiotic therapy and is recommended in COPD exacerbations associated with purulent secretions. Antibiotic therapy is directed against likely organisms (e.g. *Haemophilus influenza, Streptococcus pneumoniae, Moraxella catarrhalis*) and adjusted according to microbiological results. Initial empirical therapy should be with an aminopenicillin, a macrolide or a tetracycline.
- **Theophyllines**: these should only be used as an adjunct if the response to nebulised bronchodilators is inadequate. To prevent toxicity, plasma theophylline levels should be measured within 24 h of starting therapy and interactions with other drugs reviewed.
- **Respiratory stimulants**: these are only appropriate when non-invasive ventilation is not available.

Ventilatory Support

Non-invasive Positive Pressure Ventilation

Non-invasive positive pressure ventilation (NIPPV) has repeatedly been shown to be effective in the management of persistent hypercapnic ventilatory failure occurring during severe exacerbations of COPD despite optimal medical therapy. It is most effectively delivered by well-trained staff in an appropriate setting (e.g. HDU). **Selection criteria**: for NIPPV include severe dyspnoea, moderate to severe acidosis (pH 7.3–7.35) and hypercapnia ($PaCO_2$ 6–8 kPa) and respiratory rate >25 breaths/min. **Exclusion criteria**: include cardiovascular instability, impaired consciousness, respiratory arrest, lack of cooperation, high risk of aspiration, facial surgery or other factors preventing application of facemasks.

Three recent systematic reviews report a reduction in endotracheal intubation rates and in-hospital mortality in hypercapnic COPD exacerbations treated with NIPPV. Although one suggested that the benefit was limited to more severe cases (pH < 7.3), this was not supported by the most recent publication. As compared to standard treatment alone, NIPPV is associated with quicker improvement in pH, $PaCO_2$, respiratory rate and breathlessness, resulting in a 28% reduction in endotracheal intubation rate, a 10% reduction in mortality rate and a 4–6-day reduction in hospital stay. Most of the studies have included highly selected COPD cases with moderate respiratory failure (pH < 7.35; $PaCO_2$ 6–8 kPa, respiratory rate > 25 breaths/min) and have demonstrated failure rates of 20–30% as judged by death or the requirement for endotracheal intubation. Most studies report that response in the first 2 h of NIPPV (as measured by improvement in pH and $PaCO_2$) is predictive of success or failure. Higher failure rates (35–49%) have been reported in series of less carefully selected patients.

Mechanical Ventilation

Mechanical ventilation (MV) may be lifesaving in COPD exacerbations, but whenever possible should be avoided because (a) most patients without advanced cor pulmonale tolerate hypoxaemia and acidosis well; (b) spontaneously breathing patients have an effective cough; (c) COPD patients are at particularly high risk of developing ventilator-associated complications (e.g. barotrauma, pneumothorax, infection, hypotension); and (d) weaning can be difficult due to respiratory muscle weakness and the associated increase in work of breathing associated with hyperinflation (Figures 3.2 and 3.3). **Indications for MV**: include severe hypoxaemia ($PaO_2 < 5.3\,kPa$), respiratory rate > 35 breaths/min, increasing acidosis (pH < 7.25), hypercapnia ($PaCO_2 > 8\,kPa$), respiratory arrest, NIPPV failure, confusion, poor cough and haemodynamic instability. *Mortality* in ventilated COPD patients is about 20%, with higher mortality in those requiring > 72 h MV (37%) and those who fail an extubation attempt (36%). Mean duration of ventilation is between 5 and 9 days. Contrary to general opinion, mortality in ventilated COPD patients with respiratory failure is less than that in non-COPD cases.

In end-stage COPD with reduced exercise tolerance, resting breathlessness and loss of independence it may be appropriate to limit ventilatory support to NIPPV. The decision not to ventilate should be based on health status and an estimate of survival time based on previous functional status, BMI, LTOT requirement when well, co-morbidities and previous ICU admissions. Neither age nor FEV_1 should be used in isolation when assessing suitability for MV. A clear statement of the patients' wishes in the form of an advance directive or 'living-will' always makes these difficult decisions easier.

Mechanical ventilation in COPD (and asthma) is associated with specific problems (Figures 3.2 and 3.3):

1. *'Dynamic' hyperinflation and associated auto-PEEP*: these may occur when expiratory time is inadequate (rapid ventilatory rates) or tidal volumes are too high. The adverse consequences include increased work of breathing, haemodynamic instability and patient–ventilator dysynchrony. Barotrauma is an obvious risk of serious hyperinflation. Unlike restrictive disease, obstructive airways disease allows good transmission of alveolar pressure to the pleural space, and the haemodynamic effects of auto-PEEP may be more severe than those caused by similar levels of physician-applied PEEP. Cardiac output may fall during intubation and cardiopulmonary resuscitation, as air trapping associated with vigorous ventilation impairs venous return. Auto-PEEP also adds to the work of breathing by presenting an increased threshold load to inspiration, impairing inspiratory muscle strength and by depressing the trigger sensitivity of the ventilator. Addition of low levels of PEEP (less than auto-PEEP) effectively replaces the auto-PEEP, improving comfort, reducing work of breathing and marginally improving distribution of ventilation without increasing hyperinflation. *Management*: ventilated COPD patients must be checked at intervals for evidence of dynamic hyperinflation. If present, bronchodilation, increased expiratory time (i.e. decreased respiratory rate), reduced tidal ventilation and setting PEEP at a similar level to auto-PEEP all reduce dynamic hyperinflation and its associated effects.

2. *Metabolic alkalosis*: avoid over-ventilating patients with long-standing CO_2 retention as this may cause metabolic alkalosis.

3. *Discontinuation of MV (weaning)*: cautious weaning is undertaken as soon as possible, but can be difficult and hazardous in COPD patients. The best method is debated, but whether pressure support or a T-piece trial is used, weaning is shortened when a clinical protocol is adopted. Several recent trials indicate that NIPPV can facilitate and shorten the weaning process in COPD patients with acute or chronic respiratory failure[12]. Compared with invasive pressure support ventilation, NIPPV during weaning shortened weaning time, reduced ICU length of stay, decreased nosocomial pneumonia and improved survival rates.

Discharge After COPD Exacerbation

Prior to discharge patients must be clinically stable, with stable oximetry and blood gases, re-established on their optimal maintenance bronchodilator therapy, with appropriate support for discharge (e.g. education, oxygen delivery, visiting nurse). Arrangements for follow-up should have been made.

References

1. National clinical guideline on management of chronic obstructive pulmonary disease in adults in primary and secondary care (NICE guidelines). *Thorax.* 2004;59(Suppl 1):1–232. Available at: www.nice.org.uk/CG0 12niceguideline. Access data February 2004.

2. Celli BR, MacNee W and the ATS/ERS Task Force. Standards for the diagnosis and treatment of patients

with COPD: a summary of the ATS/ERS position paper. *Eur Respir J.* 2004;23:932–946. Available at: www.ersnet.org. Access data October 2004.

3. Global strategy for the diagnosis, management and prevention of chronic obstructive pulmonary disease; NHLBI/WHO workshop report (GOLD guidelines) NIH Publication No. 2701A. Available at: www.goldcopd.com. Accessed March 2001.

4. The COPD Guidelines Group of the Standards of Care Committee of the BTS: BTS guidelines for the management of chronic obstructive pulmonary disease. *Thorax.* 1997;52(Suppl 5):S1–28.

5. ATS guidelines: Standards for the diagnosis and care of patients with chronic obstructive pulmonary disease. Am J Respir Crit Case 1995;152:S77–S120. Available at: www.thoracie.org. 1995.

6. Cooper CB, Tashkin DP. Recent developments in inhaled therapy in stable chronic obstructive pulmonary disease. *BMJ.* 2005;330:640–644.

7. Calverly PMA, Koulouris NG. Flow limitation and dynamic hyperinflation: key concepts in modern respiratory physiology. *Eur Respir J.* 2005;25:186–199.

8. O'Donnell DE, Fluge T, Gerken F, et al. Effects of tiotropium on lung hyperinflation, dyspnoea, and exercise tolerance in COPD. *Eur Respir J.* 2004;23:832–840.

9. Barnes PJ, Stockley RA. COPD: current therapeutic interventions and future approaches. *Eur Respir J.* 2005;25:1084–1106.

10. Ram F, Picot J, Lightowler J, Wedzicha J. Non-invasive positive pressure ventilation for the treatment of respiratory failure due to exacerbations of chronic obstructive pulmonary disease. *Cochrane Database Syst Rev 1.* 2004;CD004104.

11. Calfee CS, Matthay MA. Recent advances in mechanical ventilation. *Am J Med.* 2005;118:584–591.

12. Nava S, Ambrosino N, Clini E, et al. Noninvasive mechanical ventilation in the weaning of patients with respiratory failure due to chronic obstructive pulmonary disease. A randomised controlled trial. *Ann Intern Med.* 1998;128:721–728.

4
Diffuse Interstitial Lung Disease

Aimee Brame and Andrew Jones

Abstract Patients with diffuse interstitial lung disease (DILD) admitted to the intensive care unit (ICU) often present with difficult diagnostic and management challenges to the intensivist and hence it is essential that a multidisciplinary approach is employed. Clinically, the difficulty lies in differentiating between progression of an existing DILD and the potential need for a new or increased immunosuppression, and other causes of respiratory deterioration which may require individual therapy and a potential reduction in immunosuppression. In this chapter we review the importance of the clinical history, radiological imaging and the role of additional invasive diagnostic techniques including bronchscopy, bronchoalveolar lavage and transbronchial versus open surgical biopsy, in complex patients. We review both disease-specific and general critical care management for such patients including the limited role of lung transplantation. In the absence of a reversible disease, the prognosis for patients with DILD requiring mechanical ventilation is extremely poor, and the importance of effective palliation and end-of-life-care management is discussed.

Introduction

The differential diagnosis of diffuse interstitial lung disease (DILD) is extremely broad, encompassing a wide range of lung pathologies, due to a large number of aetiological causes (Table 4.1). In addition, an individual disease may result in differing clinical and histopathological presentations, this being particularly important in connective tissue-related DILD. Importantly, some DILDs are more responsive to immunosuppressive therapy and hence have a better prognosis. Given the complexity of the diagnosis and subsequent management, it is essential that a multidisciplinary approach, potentially involving respiratory physicians, radiologists, microbiologists, thoracic surgeons and histopathologists is employed in the diagnosis and subsequent management of patients with DILD in the intensive care unit (ICU).[1,2]

Clinical Presentation

Rarely the first presentation of DILD may result in acute respiratory failure. In the absence of specific clinical history or findings, such patients are often treated as for pulmonary infection, with failure of resolution, or ongoing deterioration being the stimulus to challenge the diagnosis. A high index of suspicion, a thorough, directed history and examination, with early involvement of a respiratory physician are vital to minimize delay in such cases.

More commonly, it is the development of respiratory failure on a background of established DILD that first brings the patient to the attention of the ICU team. Clinically, the differential diagnosis usually lies between a deterioration in the underlying disease requiring increased immunosuppression, and other causes of respiratory deterioration (infection, pulmonary embolus, heart failure), which may require additional therapy and possibly a reduction in immunosuppression. This

TABLE 4.1. Recognised causes of diffuse interstitial lung disease

Occupational/environmental	
Non-organic	
Asbestosis	
Silicosis	
Coal workers pneumoconiosis	
Organic	
Hypersensitivity pneumonitis, e.g. Bird fancier's lung, Farmer's lung	
Collagen vascular disease	
Rheumatoid arthritis	
Poly/dermatomyositis	
Scleroderma	
Primary Sjogren's syndrome	
Systemic lupus erythematosis	
Ankylosing spondylitis	
Vasculitis-related	
Wegeners granulomatosis	
Churg–Strauss vasculitis	
Pauci immune vasculitis	
Goodpature's syndrome (anti-GBM disease)	
Drug-related	
Amiodarone	Cyclophosphamide
Sulphasalazine	Chlorambucil
Gold	Mephalan
Penicillamine	Methotrexate
Mitomycin	Azothioprine
Bleomycin	Cytosine arabinoside
Busulfan	Nitrofurantoin
Physical agents	
Radiation/radiotherapy	
Cocaine inhalation	
Intravenous drug abuse	
Paraquat toxicity	
Neoplastic disease	
Bronchoalveolar cell carcinoma	
Lymphangitis carcinomatosis	
Pulmonary lymphoma	
Circulatory disorders	
Pulmonary oedema	
Pulmonary veno-occlusive disease	
Chronic infection	
Tuberculosis	
Fungal disease (aspergillosis, histoplasmosis)	
Miscellaneous	
Sarcoidosis	
Amyloidosis	
Alveolar proteinosis	
Chronic aspiration	
Eosinophilic pneumonia	
Idiopathic interstitial pneumonias	
Acute interstitial pneumonia (AIP)	
Usual interstitial pneumonitis (UIP)	
Desquamative interstitial pneumonitis (DIP)	
Non-specific interstitial pneumonia (NSIP)	
Organizing pneumonia (OP)	
Respiratory bronchiolitis interstitial lung disease (RBILD)	

distinction is difficult in such patients because the clinical presentations may overlap.

Unfortunately, in the majority of the connective tissue diseases and other forms of DILD, there is no serological marker that closely correlates with pulmonary disease activity. In addition, commonly used laboratory indices of infection (e.g. white blood cell count, erythrocyte sedimentation rate, C-reactive protein), may be influenced by the underlying connective tissue disease, or its treatment (immunosuppressive agents), and therefore lack sensitivity or specificity. The situation is further complicated with the development of multi-organ dysfunction and increased risks of nosocomial infection, in patients requiring intensive care. New markers designed to differentiate infection from inflammation (e.g. procalcitonin) have been shown to perform well in clinical studies, including both the critical care population and in patients with systemic autoimmune disease, but are not widely available for clinical use.[3,4]

Investigation

Given the severity of illness with which these patients present, a multidisciplinary and calibrated diagnostic approach is recommended (Figure 4.2).

Radiological Investigation

In this group of patients the importance of reviewing available prior imaging, to place present findings in perspective to established disease, and to develop temporal relationships, cannot be understated. That said, unfortunately chest radiography may be unhelpful in distinguishing pulmonary infection from progression of DILD in the ICU population.[5] Computed tomography, in particular high-resolution computed tomography (HRCT), is now central to the diagnosis and management of diffuse interstitial lung disease.[1] It has been shown to be a safe method of obtaining clinical and physiological information in the critically ill,[6] and may be diagnostic in advanced DILD[7] obviating the need for invasive investigation. Although characteristic HRCT patterns are described for specific forms of DILD and some infections (Figure 4.1a–c), CT scanning has not

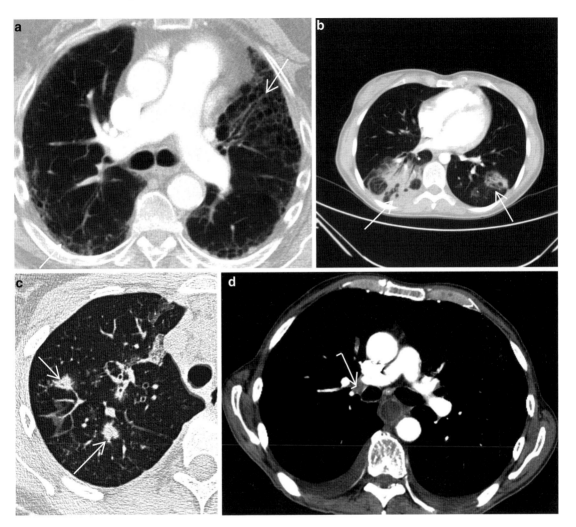

FIGURE 4.1. (a) Sub-pleural fibrosis (Lower 7 O'clock arrow corresponds to sub-pleural change) with marked honeycomb change (Upper 1 O'clock arrow corresponds to honey-comb lung). Typical of UIP which is typically poorly responsive to therapy. (b) Multifocal (often peri-bronchial) consolidation (arrows) compatible with infection, but in this case represented organizing pneumonia which is potentially reversible with immunosuppression. This image also highlights the use of CT in identifying sites for further sampling (BAL or biopsy). (c) Mutiple medium-sized nodules with a halo of ground glass shadowing, highly suggestive of fungal infection (arrows). (d) CT pulmonary angiogram (CTPA) with filling defect/thrombus occluding right lower lobe pulmonary artery (arrow).

been evaluated as a diagnostic test for opportunistic infection in the ventilated patient with DILD. Poor quality images can be a major constraint in the breathless and ventilated patient, along with other technical issues and interpretation with an experienced radiologist is recommended. HRCT can usually be combined with CT pulmonary angiography if pulmonary embolic disease is under consideration as a cause for clinical deterioration (Figure 4.1d). In addition, if inconclusive itself, CT may define the optimal site for further investigation (e.g. bronchoalveolar lavage [BAL] or biopsy).

Microbiological Investigation

The spectrum of potential infective organisms is dependent on a number of factors including: presence of neutropenia[8] level and type of immunosuppressive therapy,[9,10] prior administration of empirical antimicrobial therapy[11] and timing relative to hospital admission and onset of

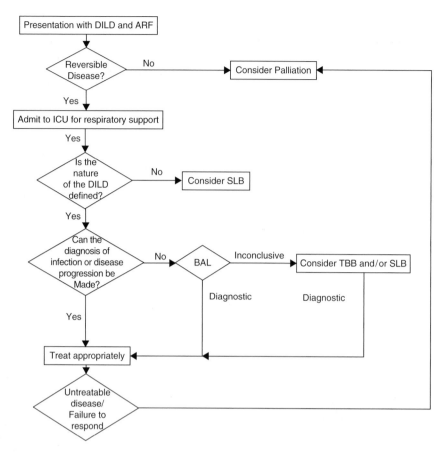

FIGURE 4.2. An algorithm for the management of patients with diffuse interstitial lung disease (DILD) and acute respiratory failure (ARF). Abbreviations: BAL, bronchoalveolar lavage; TBB, transbronchial biopsy; SLB, surgical lung biopsy.

mechanical ventilation.[12,13] Although their exact incidence varies between series, in the non-HIV positive immunocompromised patient, the commonest infectious pathogens are bacterial (~40%), followed by fungal (~30%), viral (~20%), *Pneumocystis jiroveci* (~10%) and *Mycobacterium tuberculosis* (<5%)—with mixed pathogens occurring commonly (~20%).

Routine specimens should include blood cultures, sputum (gram stain, fungal smears, culture), urinary antigen detection (Pneumococcus, Legionella), nasal pharyngeal aspirate or swabs (or BAL see below) for respiratory virus direct fluorescent antibody (DFA) testing and culture, CMV antigenaemia and serum PCR. In less sick patients with mild hypoxaemia, induced sputum (mycobacteria, pneumocystis) should be considered, but is usually superseded by bronchoscopy and BAL in sicker individuals.

Ordinarily, bronchoscopy with BAL plays a relatively minor role in the clinical management of DILD. However, in the clinical scenario of pulmonary infiltrates in the setting of immunosuppression, BAL can be crucial in the detection of opportunistic infection as well as non-infective causes of diffuse alveolar shadowing such as alveolar haemorrhage and malignancy.[14,15] Although bacterial pathogens are the most commonly isolated, diagnostic testing should aim to exclude atypical, opportunistic, fungal, mycobacterial and viral infections along the lines discussed above. New diagnostic techniques applicable to BAL fluid include antigen detection (e.g. *Aspergillous* spp., *Cryptococcus neoformans*, *Legionella pneumophila*), antibody detection (anti-pneumolysin in detection of pneumococcal pneumonia), special methods for culture (BACTEC radiometric culture for mycobacteria), as well as molecular biological techniques such as the polymerise chain reaction (PCR) (e.g. CMV, *Herpes simplex*, *M. tuberculosis*).[16] However, the clinical usefulness of these tests is yet to be validated, and likely to be highly dependent on the quality of the specimen, BAL technique and population studied. Clinicians are advised to seek early microbiological advice regarding their use in such patients.

If adequate precautions are taken, bronchoscopy with BAL has been shown to be safe in immuno-suppressed patients, including those with haematological dysfunction[17] and critically ill patients requiring mechanical ventilation.[18] However, deterioration in respiratory mechanics and gas exchange is well recognised.[19,20] Therefore, in self-ventilating patients who are at high risk of requiring mechanical ventilation,[21] the additional diagnostic benefits need to be carefully considered and thought given to whether the procedure should be performed in the ICU.

Lung Biopsy

If BAL is unhelpful, attention often turns to more invasive methods of tissue sampling, that is, transbronchial biopsy (TBB) or surgical lung biopsy (SLB). The added value of TBB in patients undergoing BAL remains contentious. However, in a retrospective evaluation in both HIV and non-HIV immunosuppressed patients TBB was more sensitive than BAL (77% vs 48% in HIV disease, 55% vs 20% in haematological malignancy, 57% vs 27% in renal transplant recipients) and there were few serious complications.[22] In patients with HIV infection it has been argued that a negative BAL result should prompt a repeat BAL with TBB at the most abnormal site; this approach has a diagnostic yield of 90% for nodules or focal infiltrates.[23] A similar approach has been found to be successful and safe in mechanically ventilated patients.[24,25] In one small retrospective review ($n = 38$), a combined procedure allowed a diagnosis in 74% of patients, resulting in a confirmation of clinical diagnosis in 11% and therapeutic modification in 63%. Complications included pneumothorax (24%), mild haemorrhage (11%) and transient hypotension (5%), but there were no serious complications or deaths. When BAL and TBB are non-diagnostic, SLB via either a mini-thoracotomy or video-assisted thoracoscopy (VATS) may be considered. Although widely accepted in DILD in general, the role of SLB has been questioned in ventilated subjects because of a perception of higher risk and reduced benefit in critically ill patients. The diagnostic yield of SLB in ventilated patients varies from 46% to 100%.[26-29] Perceived benefits of increased diagnostic accuracy include: confirmation of the diagnosis and continuation of existing therapy, initiation or increase of immunosuppression, alterations in antimicrobial therapy, withdrawal of unnecessary medication and, where the underlying disease is untreatable, allowing the focus of care to change to more palliative goals. However, in most studies such therapeutic modification does not reliably affect outcome. Although major complications or death directly related to the procedure are uncommon, 'minor' complications are reported in 20–50%, with persistent air leaks being the most pertinent in the ventilated patient. Factors predicting mortality in ventilated patients with pulmonary infiltrates undergoing SLB have included an immunocompromised status at the onset of respiratory failure or current immunosuppressive treatment, severe hypoxia, multi-organ failure and old age.[26-30]

Given the high hospital mortality and poor long-term prognosis in such patients, others have argued that if broad-spectrum antibiotic cover (including cotrimoxazole to cover PCP), and corticosteroids are included in empirical therapeutic trials, then SLB is of limited additional clinical benefit in this population of patients.[31,32]

Treatment

In cases where an alternative diagnosis is found, this should be treated along standard lines.

Antimicrobial Therapy

Given the considerations discussed above, it is usually important to commence early, effective empiric antimicrobial therapy based on existing clinical and microbiological information prior to the results of more immediate investigations. Invariably, broad-spectrum antibiotic, and often antifungal and antiviral, therapy is commenced pending the results of BAL and CT—with rationalisation of therapy once results become available. Direct involvement of a microbiologist is advised.

Immunosuppressive Therapy

Where increased disease activity is suspected, and usually following the exclusion of infection, then consideration needs to be given to initiation/further increases in immunosuppression. In the absence of randomized controlled trials, corticosteroids are the mainstay of therapy with initial doses of 0.5–1.0 mg/kg of prednisolone equivalent being usual, the variation being partly dependent on the underlying diagnosis. In patients with severe or rapidly progressive disease, or those receiving mechanical ventilation for acute respiratory failure, some centres, including our own, would initiate therapy with 3 days of intravenous methyprednisolone (0.5–1 g daily). In severe cases, or those not responsive to corticosteroid therapy, adjunct agents are sometimes employed, most commonly cyclophosphamide (0.5–1.0 g/m^2 BSA), with dose adjustment for renal function, age and obesity. In patients with an adequate renal function promotion of a good urine output (>100 mL/h) and continuous catheter drainage should be adequate to avoid complications of haemorrhagic cystitis, if there is concern the adjunctive use of MESNA is recommended.

No strong evidence exists for these more aggressive immunosuppressive regimens, which are extrapolated from experience in other disciplines. As such we would advise that they should be undertaken only in partnership with specialist clinicians familiar with their use in the wider setting. Of particular concern, is the risk of nosocomial infection, and appropriate measures should be taken to minimize this. In addition, use of immunosuppression may prompt the need for antimicrobial prophylaxis (PCP, TB, CMV etc.).

Critical Care Supportive Therapy

Non-invasive ventilation (NIV) has been shown to avert the need for intubation and decrease the likelihood of nosocomial infection in chronic obstructive pulmonary disease, acute pulmonary oedema and in some cases of respiratory failure associated with immunosuppression.[33] In the setting of pulmonary fibrosis, NIV is an option in mild respiratory failure, but we recommend that it is employed in an appropriate setting given the potential for deterioration and requirement for invasive ventilation.

The onset of severe respiratory failure and/or multi-organ dysfunction may prompt a multidisciplinary discussion regarding the benefits of ongoing ICU support versus a more palliative approach. If ongoing support is deemed appropriate, then it should occur in line with proposed evidence-based guidelines.[34] Although there is little evidence for specific ventilatory strategies for patients with DILD, our approach is to extrapolate present guidelines for acute lung injury,[35] limiting excessive tidal volume and pressure changes and accepting modest degrees of 'permissive' hypoxaemia and hypercapnia until the patient responds to a specific treatment. Given the lack of evidence of long-term benefit, with worsening gas exchange, adjunctive therapies such as inhaled vasodilators, prone positioning and high frequency oscillatory ventilation should be applied on an individual patient basis.

Lung Transplantation

Mechanical ventilation has been traditionally regarded as a strong relative contraindication to lung transplantation due to concerns about airway microbial colonisation and subsequent risk of pneumonia, the effects of long-term immobility and severe muscular deconditioning and other complications associated with mechanical ventilation (e.g. sepsis, deep venous thrombosis, gastrointestinal haemorrhage, altered gut motility and nutritional problems etc.).[36] Individual successes have been documented, but data reported to the International Society of Heart Lung Transplantation/United Network for Organ Sharing indicate a threefold increase in 1-year mortality compared to non-ventilated recipients.[37] It has been suggested that a distinction should be made between stable, chronically ventilator-dependent patients and those with acute respiratory failure. In a recent retrospective review of transplantation in 21 ventilator-dependent patients, 3 of 5 unstable patients died shortly after transplantation, compared with 0 of 16 stable ventilator-dependent patients. The 5-year actuarial survival rate of 40% in the latter group was comparable to that seen in non-ventilated individuals in the transplant program.[38] However, given the scarcity of donor organs, the indications for transplantation in those receiving mechanical ventilation remain imprecise and controversial. Such decisions should be individualized, with decisions based on variables such as, the type and activity of the underlying DILD, the reversibility of any superimposed process and the likelihood of expeditious transplantation. Transplantation during the acute episode is seldom practical and unlikely to be successful.

Outcome

When considering outcome in this patient group, several limitations have to be recognized. Firstly, all studies are retrospective reviews from single centers. Secondly, most cover periods before the more stringent classification of these diseases and have therefore concentrated on 'idiopathic pulmonary fibrosis'—considered to be resistant to therapy and irreversible in most patients. Finally, the spectrum in response of these diseases to immunosuppressive therapy needs to be borne in mind when making decisions in individual patients. Accepting these considerations the overall outlook for patients with established or progressive interstitial lung disease receiving mechanical ventilation is grave.[39–43]

End-of-Life Care

Given this grave prognosis, we advocate that this group of patients be considered for a 'trial of ICU'[44] in the hope of identifying a treatable cause for their deterioration, such as acute exacerbation of the underlying disease, infection, heart failure or pulmonary embolism. However, in the absence of any reversible element, progression despite treatment or the progression to multi-organ failure suggests that further escalation or prolonged life support may be inappropriate. Under such circumstances the goals of therapy may switch to palliation, including the option of treatment withdrawal. Recent guidelines advocate a shared approach to end-of-life decision making, including the patient (as appropriate), their family and the multidisciplinary team.[45, 46] Patient comfort becomes paramount, and all therapies need to be reassessed with this goal in mind. Those that do not add benefit should be discontinued, and levels of some existing therapies, e.g. analgesia, anti-emetics may need to be increased. Normal ICU practice may need to be reassessed, e.g. patient monitoring, routine interventions and investigations, with particular attention to the patient's privacy, family and spiritual needs. Withdrawal of life support measures should be undertaken by experienced staff with knowledge of how to anticipate and address potential issues for the deteriorating patient and their family.

Summary

- Diagnosis and management of DILD in patients on the ICU is complex and requires a multidisciplinary approach from the outset.
- Often management is directed at distinguishing between exacerbation of the underlying DILD and superadded complications which are predominantly infective in origin.
- DILD includes a spectrum of diseases with variable responses to immunosuppressive therapy, knowledge that needs to be factored in to an individual patient's management on the ICU.
- In the absence of reversible pathology, the prognosis for mechanically ventilated patients is extremely poor, and careful attention should be given to end-of-life care issues.

Abbreviations

BAL	Broncho-alveolar lavage
BSA	Body surface area
CMV	Cytomegalovirus
CT	Computed tomography
CTPA	Computed tomography pulmonary angiography
CXR	Chest x-ray
DILD	Diffuse interstitial lung disease
HRCT	High resolution computed tomography
ICU	Intensive care unit
PCP	Pnemocystis pneumonia
PCR	Polymerise chain reaction
SLB	Surgical lung biopsy
TB	Tuberculosis
TBB	Trans-bronchial biopsy
VATS	Video-assisted thoracoscopic surgery

References

1. American Thoracic Society. Idiopathic pulmonary fibrosis: diagnosis and treatment. International consensus statement. American Thoracic Society (ATS),

and the European Respiratory Society (ERS). *Am J Respir Crit Care Med.* 2000;161:646–664.

2. British Thoracic Society. BTS guidelines on the diagnosis, assessment and treatment of diffuse parenchymal lung disease in adults. *Thorax.* 1999;54(Suppl 1): S4–14.

3. Brunkhorst R, Eberhardt OK, Haubitz M, Brunkhorst FM. Procalcitonin for discrimination of systemic autoimmune disease and systemic bacterial infection. *Intensive Care Med.* 2000;26:S199–201.

4. Becker KL, Snider R, Nylen ES (2008) Procalcitonin assay in systemic inflammation, infection, and sepsis: clinical utility and limitations. *Crit Care Med.* 2008;36:941–952.

5. Hansell DM. Imaging the injured lung. In: Evans TW, Haslett C, eds. *Acute Respiratory Distress in Adults.* London: Chapman & Hall; 1996:361–379.

6. Pesenti A, Tagliabue P, Patroniti N, Fumagalli R. Computerised tomography scan imaging in acute respiratory distress syndrome. *Intensive Care Med.* 2001;27:631–639.

7. Primack SL, Hartman TE, Hansell DM, Müller N. End stage lung disease: findings in 61 patients. *Radiology.* 1993;189:681–686.

8. Cordonnier C, Escudier E, Verra F, Brochard L, Bernaudin JF, Fleury-Feith J. Bronchoalveolar lavage during neutropenic episodes: diagnostic yield and cellular pattern. *Eur Respir J.* 1994;7:114–120.

9. Ewig S, Torres A, Riquelme R, et al. Pulmonary complications inpatients with haematological malignancies treated at a respiratory ICU. *Eur Respir J.* 1998;12:116–122.

10. Dunagan DP, Baker AM, Hurd DD, Haponik EF. Bronchoscopic evaluation of pulmonary infiltrates following bone marrow transplantation. *Chest.* 1997;111:135–141.

11. Hohenadel IA, Kiworr M, Genitsariotis R, et al. Role of bronchoalveolar lavage in immunocompromised patients with pneumonia treated with broad spectrum antibiotic and antifungal regimen. *Thorax.* 2001;56:115–120.

12. Fagon J, Chastre J, Wolf M, et al. Invasive and non-invasive strategies for management of suspected ventilator-associated pneumonia. *Ann Intern Med.* 2000;132:621–630.

13. Mehta R, Niederman MS. Adequate empirical therapy minimizes the impact of diagnostic methods in patients with ventilator-associated pneumonia. *Crit Care Med.* 2000;28:3092–3094.

14. Stover DE, Zaman MB, Hajdu SI, et al. Bronchoalveolar lavage in the diagnosis of diffuse pulmonary infiltrates in the immunocompromised host. *Ann Intern Med.* 1984;101:1–7.

15. Cordonnier C, Escudier E, Verra F, et al. Bronchoalveolar lavage during neutropenic episodes: diagnostic yield and cellular pattern. *Eur Respir J.* 1994;7:114–120.

16. Mayaud C, Cadranel J. A persistent challenge: the diagnosis of respiratory disease in the non-AIDS immunocompromised host. Thorax. 2000;55:511–517.

17. Saito H, Anaissie EJ, Morice RC, et al. Bronchoalveolar lavage in the diagnosis of pulmonary infiltrates in patients with acute leukaemia. *Chest.* 1988;94:745–749.

18. Steinberg KP, Mitchel DR, Maunder RJ, et al. Safety of bronchoalveolar lavage in patients with adult respiratory distress syndrome. *Am Rev Respir Dis.* 1993;148:556–561.

19. Montravers P, Gauzit R, Dombret MC, et al. Cardiopulmonary effects of bronchoalveolar lavage in critically ill patients. *Chest.* 1993;106:1541–1547.

20. Klein U, Karzai W, Zimmermann P, et al. Changes in pulmonary mechanics after fibreoptic bronchoalveolar lavage in mechanically ventilated patients. *Intensive Care Med.* 1998;12:1289–1293.

21. Azoulay E, Mokart D, Rabbat A et al. Diagnostic bronchoscopy in hematology and oncology patients with acute respiratory failure: prospective multicenter data. *Crit Care Med.* 2008;36:100–107.

22. Cazzadori A, Di Perri G, Todeschini G, et al. Transbronchial biopsy in the diagnosis of pulmonary infiltrates in immunocompromised patients. *Chest.* 1995;107:101–106.

23. Cadranel J, Gillet-Juvin K, Antoine M et al. Site directed bronchoalveolar lavage and transbronchial biopsy in HIV-infected patients with pneumonia. *Am J Respir Crit Care Med.* 1995;152:1103–1106.

24. O'Brien JD, Ettinger NA, Shevlin D, et al. Safety and yield of transbroncial biopsy in mechanically ventilated patients. *Crit Care Med.* 1997;25:440–446.

25. Bulpa PA, Dive AM, Mertens L et al. Combined bronchoalveolar lavage and transbronchial lung biopsy: safety and yield in ventilated patients. *Eur Respir J.* 2003;21:489–494.

26. Canver CC, Menttzer RM. The role of open lung biopsy in early and late survival of ventilator-dependent patients with diffuse idiopathic lung disease. *J Cardiovasc Surg.* 1994;35:151–155.

27. Flabouris A, Myburgh J The utility of open lung biopsy in patients requiring mechanical ventilation. *Chest.* 1999;115:811–817.

28. Warner DO, Warner MA, Divertie MB, et al. Open lung biopsy in patients with diffuse pulmonary infiltrates and acute respiratory failure. *Am Rev Respir Dis.* 1988;137: 90–94.

29. Lim SY, Suh GY, Choi JC, et al. Usefulness of open lung biopsy in mechanically ventilated patients with undiagnosed diffuse pulmonary infiltrates: influence of comorbidities and organ dysfunction. *Crit Care.* 2007;11: R93.

30. Poe RH, Wahl GW, Qazi R, et al. Predictors of mortality in the immunocompromised patient with pulmonary infiltrates. *Arch Intern Med*. 1986;146:1304–1308.

31. Potter D, Pass HI, Brower S, et al. Prospective randomized study of open lung biopsy versus empirical antibiotic therapy for acute pneumonitis in nonneutropenic cancer patients. *Ann Thorac Surg*. 1985;40:422–428.

32. McKenna RJ, Mountain CF, McMurtrey MJ. Open lung biopsy in immunocompromised patients. *Chest*. 1984;86:671–674.

33. Evans TW, Albert RK, Angus DC, et al. International Consensus Conferences in Intensive Care Medicine: Noninvasive positive pressure ventilation in acute respiratory failure. *Am J Respir Crit Care Med*. 2001;163:283–291.

34. Dellinger RP, Levy MM, Carlet JM, et al. Surviving Sepsis Campaign: International guidelines for management of severe sepsis and septic shock. *Crit Care Med*. 2008;36:296–327.

35. The Acute Respiratory Distress Syndrome Network. Ventilation with lower tidal volumes as compared with traditional tidal volumes for acute lung injury and the acute respiratory distress syndrome. *N Engl J Med*. 2000;342:1301–1308.

36. American Thoracic Society. International guidelines for the selection of lung transplant candidates. *Am J Respir Crit Care Med*. 1998;158:335–339.

37. O'Brien GD, Criner GJ. Mechanical ventilation as a bridge to lung transplantation. *J Heart Lung Transplant*. 1999;18:255–265.

38. Meyers BF, Lynch JP, Battafarano RJ, et al. Lung transplant is warranted in stable, ventilator-dependent patients. *Ann Thorac Surg*. 2000;70:1675–1678.

39. Fumeaux T, Rothmeier C, Jolliet P. Outcome of mechanical ventilation for acute respiratory failure in patients with pulmonary fibrosis. *Intensive Care Med*. 2000;12:1868–1874.

40. Stern JB, Mal H, Groussard O et al. Prognosis of patients with advanced idiopathic pulmonary fibrosis requiring mechanical ventilation for acute respiratory failure. *Chest*. 2001;120:213–219.

41. Blivet S, Philit F, Sab JM, et al. Outcome of patients with idiopathic pulmonary fibrosis admitted to the ICU for respiratory failure. *Chest*. 2001;120: 209–212.

42. Al-Hameed FM, Sharma S. Outcome of patients admitted to the intensive care unit for acute exacerbation of idiopathic pulmonary fibrosis. *Can Respir J*. 2004;11:117–122.

43. Saydain G, Islam A, Afessa B, et al. Outcome of patients with idiopathic pulmonary fibrosis admitted to the intensive care unit. *Am J Respir Crit Care Med*. 2002;166: 839–842.

44. Lecuyer L, Chevret S, Thiery G et al. The ICU trial: a new admission policy for cancer patients requiring mechanical ventilation. *Crit Care Med*. 2007;35:808–814.

45. Truog RD, Cist AF, Brackett SE, et al. Recommendations for end-of-life care in the intensive care unit: The Ethics Committee of the Society of Critical Care Medicine. *Crit Care Med*. 2001;29: 2332–2348.

46. Challenges in End-of Life Care in the USA: Statement of the 5th International Consensus Conference in Critical Care: Brussels, Belgium, April 2003: Executive Summary. *Crit Care Med*. 2004;32: 1781–1784.

5
Pneumonia

Richard Leach

Abstract Despite antibiotic therapy, pneumonia remains a significant worldwide cause of morbidity and mortality. The term pneumonia covers several distinct clinical entities, and correct classification is vital as the aetiology, infective organism, antibiotic management and outcome are determined by how and where pneumonia was contracted. Early recognition and appropriate treatment improve outcome. Critical care physicians must be familiar with all aspects of pneumonia, as they will be expected to advise on and manage severe community-acquired pneumonia (CAP), hospital-acquired pneumonia (HAP) and opportunistic pneumonias in immuno-compromised patients in the wards, high dependency units (HDUs) and intensive care units (ICUs). Differences in the recently published antibiotic guidelines between the British and American Thoracic Societies are highlighted in this chapter.

General Definition of Pneumonia

Pneumonia describes an *acute lower respiratory tract (LRT) illness*, usually but not always due to *infection*, associated with *fever*, *focal chest symptoms* (*with or without clinical signs*) and *new shadowing on chest radiography* (Figure 5.1). The many infective micro-organisms and pathological insults that cause pneumonia are listed in Table 5.1.

Classification of Pneumonia

In the clinical situation, *microbiological classification* of pneumonia is not practical, since identification of the organism, even when possible, may take several days. Likewise, *anatomical* (*radiographic*) appearance (e.g. lobar pneumonia, which describes consolidation localised to one lobe; or bronchopneumonia, which describes widespread, patchy consolidation) gives little practical information about the cause, course or prognosis of the infection. The following classification is widely accepted:

- **Community-acquired pneumonia (CAP)** describes LRT infections occurring within 48 h of hospital admission in patients who have not been hospitalised for more than 14 days. The most likely infective organisms are *Streptococcus pneumoniae* (20–75%), *Mycoplasma pneumoniae* and *Chlamydia pneumoniae*.

- **Hospital-acquired (nosocomial) pneumonia (HAP)** is defined as any LRT infection developing greater than 48 h after hospital admission, which was not incubating at the time of admission. HAP includes: (i) *ventilator-associated pneumonia* (*VAP*), which refers to pneumonia developing greater than 48–72 h after endotracheal intubation; and (ii) *health-care-associated pneumonia* (*HCAP*), which includes any patient admitted to hospital for more than 2 days within 90 days of the infection, residing in a nursing home, receiving therapy (e.g. wound care, intravenous [iv] therapy) within 30 days of the current infection, or attending a hospital or haemodialysis clinic. Likely, causative organisms differ from CAP and include Gram-negative bacilli (~70%) or *Staphylococcus* (~15%).

- **Aspiration/anaerobic pneumonia** occurs due to *bacteroides* and other anaerobic infections, which follow aspiration of oropharyngeal contents due

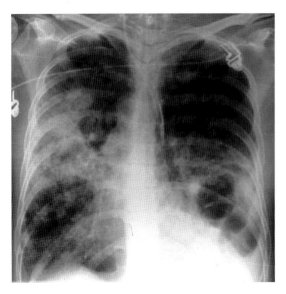

FIGURE 5.1. Pneumonia chest x-ray (CXR).

TABLE 5.1. Micro-organisms and pathological insults that cause pneumonia

Bacterial infections	Atypical infections	Fungal infection
Streptococcus pneumoniae	Mycoplasma	Aspergillus
Haemophilus influenzae	pneumoniae	Candida
Escherichia Coli	Coxiella burnetti	Nocardia
Klebsiella pneumoniae	Chlamydia psittaci	Histoplasmosis
Pseudomonas aeruginosa	Legionella	
	pneumophila	
Viral infections	**Protozoal infections**	**Others**
Influenza	Pneumocystis	Aspiration
Coxsackie	carinii	Bronchiectasis
Respiratory syncytial	Toxoplasmosis	Cystic fibrosis
Cytomegalovirus	Amoeboesis	Lipoid pneumonia
Adenovirus		Radiation

to impaired laryngeal competence (e.g. cerebrovascular accident [CVA]) or reduced consciousness (e.g. drugs, alcohol, postoperative).

- **Opportunistic pneumonia** occurs in immuno-suppressed patients taking high-dose steroids, chemotherapy or who are HIV positive. They are susceptible to viral, fungal and mycobacterial infections, in addition to the normal range of bacterial organisms.
- **Recurrent pneumonia** occurs due to aerobic and anaerobic organisms in cystic fibrosis and bronchiectasis.

Community–Acquired Pneumonia

Epidemiology: Incidence

Prospective population studies report an annual CAP incidence of 5–11 cases per 1,000 adults and ~15–45% require hospitalisation (1–4 cases per 1,000) of whom 5–10% are treated in ICU. Incidence is highest in the very young and elderly (~35 per 1,000 in patients aged >75 years). *Mortality* is <1% in patients treated at home, 5–12% in hospitalised patients and 25–50% in ICU patients. *Seasonal variation* occurs with individual pathogens; *M. pneumonia, Staphylococcus* and influenza virus occur in winter, *Legionella* spp. in September–October and *Coxiella burnetii* in spring. Annual cycles are also reported (e.g. 4 yearly *mycoplasma* epidemics). Frequent viral infections increase CAP in winter.

Aetiology

Identifying the causative pathogen in CAP is difficult and results vary with methodology (e.g. bacterial quantification), geography (e.g. the UK, Europe, the USA) and illness severity (e.g. community, hospital or ICU). No infective cause is found in 30–50% of cases, but in virtually all studies the most frequently identified organism is *S. pneumoniae* (20–75%). The 'atypical' bacterial pathogens including *M. pneumonaie, Chlamydia pneumoniae* and *Legionalla* spp. (2–25%) and viral infections including influenza A and B (8–12%) are relatively common causes of CAP. *Haemophilus influenza* and *Moraxella catarrhalis* are often associated with COPD exacerbations and staphylococcal infection may follow influenza. *Respiratory syncytial virus* affects children <2 years old. Alcoholic, diabetic, heart failure and nursing-home patients are prone to infection with staphylococcal, anaerobic and Gram-negative organisms.

Risk Factors

Table 5.2 lists factors associated with increased risk of CAP. *Specific risk factors* include *age* (e.g. mycoplasma in young adults), *occupation* (e.g. brucellosis in abattoir workers, *C. burnetii* [Q fever] in sheep workers), *environment* (e.g. psittacosis with pet birds, tularaemia and erlichiosis due to tick bites) or *geographical* (e.g. coccidomycosis

TABLE 5.2. Risk factors for pneumonia

- Age: >65, <5 years old
- Diabetes mellitus
- Chronic disease (e.g. renal, lung)
- Alcohol dependency
- Aspiration (e.g. epilepsy)
- Recent viral illness (e.g. influenza)
- Malnutrition
- Immunosuppression: (e.g. drugs, HIV)
- Environmental (e.g. psitticosis)
- Occupational (e.g. Q fever)
- Travel abroad (e.g. paragonomiasis)
- Air conditioning (e.g. Legionella)
- Mechanical ventilation
- Postoperative (e.g. obesity, smoking)

in southwest USA). Epidemics of *C. burnetti* (Q fever) or *Legionella pneumophila* are often localised. For example, patients developing Legionnaires disease may have been exposed to a contaminated air conditioner at a specific hotel.

Diagnosis

Diagnosis of CAP on the basis of history and clinical findings is inaccurate without a chest radiograph, and several studies have demonstrated that the causative organism cannot be predicted from clinical features. In particular, 'atypical' pathogens do not have a characteristic clinical presentation. The diagnostic aims are to (1) establish the *diagnosis of pneumonia*, (2) determine *classification* (*aetiology*), which aids initial antibiotic choice, (3) assess *severity*, which determines the most appropriate ward placement (e.g. ward, HDU or ICU), (4) *adjust antibiotic therapy* when microbiological results are available, and (5) identify and treat *complications*.

- **Clinical features:** *symptoms* may be general (e.g. malaise, fever, rigors, myalgia) or chest-specific (e.g. dyspnoea, pleurisy, cough, discoloured sputum, haemoptysis). *Signs* include cyanosis, tachycardia and tachypnoea; with focal dullness, crepitations, bronchial breathing and pleuritic rub on chest examination. In young or old patients and in those with atypical pneumonias (e.g. mycoplasma, legionella) *non-respiratory features* (e.g. headache, confusion, rashes, diarrhoea) may predominate. *Complications* are shown in Figure 5.3.
- **Investigations:** *routine blood tests* should be included. White cell count (WCC) and C-reactive protein (CRP) confirm infection, abnormal liver

function tests suggest *Legionella* spp. or *M. pneumoniae* infection and haemolysis and cold agglutinins occur in ~50% of mycoplasma infections. *Blood gases*: are performed to identify respiratory failure. *Microbiology*: is essential in all cases but no micro-organism is isolated in ~33–50% of patients due to previous antibiotic therapy or inadequate specimen collection. Blood cultures are recommended in severe pneumonia and may be positive in ~25%. Sputum, pleural fluid and bronchoalveolar lavage samples, with appropriate staining (e.g. Gram stain), culture and assessment of antibiotic sensitivity may determine the pathogen (~30–50%) and effective therapy. *Serology*: identifies *M. pneumoniae* infection, but long processing times limit clinical value. Recently developed rapid antigen detection tests for *Legionella* spp. (e.g. in urine) and *S. pneumoniae* (e.g. in serum, pleural fluid, urine) are more useful. *Radiological*: chest x-ray (CXR) and computed tomography (CT) scans aid diagnosis, monitor deterioration, indicate severity and aid early detection of complications (Figure 5.3). Resolution of radiological changes may be slow and should not lead to further investigation during clinical improvement.

- **Severity assessment:** the following features are associated with increased CAP mortality and indicate the need for monitoring on an HDU/ICU. (a) *Clinical*: age > 60 years, respiratory rate > 30/min, diastolic blood pressure < 60 mmHg, new atrial fibrillation, confusion, multilobar involvement and coexisting illness. (b) *Laboratory*: urea > 7 mmol/L, albumin < 35 g/L, hypoxaemia PO_2 < 8 kPa, leucopenia (WCC < 4 × 10^9/L), leucocytosis (WCC > 20 × 10^9/L) and bacteraemia. *Severity scoring*: the recently validated CURB-65 score, which allocates one points for each of confusion; urea > 7 mmol/L; respiratory rate > 30/min; low systolic (<90 mmHg) or diastolic (<60 mmHg) blood pressure and age > 65 years, stratifies patients into mortality groups suitable for different management pathways. A score greater than 4 indicates the need for admission to a monitored bed in an HDU or ICU.

Management

Supportive Measures

These include oxygen to maintain PaO_2 > 8 kPa (SaO_2 > 90%) and intravenous (iv) fluid and if necessary inotropic support to maintain a mean blood pressure > 65 mmHg and urine output 0.5–1 mL/kg/min. *Ventilatory support:* non-invasive (e.g. CPAP, NIPPV) or mechanical ventilation (MV) may be required in respiratory failure. Persisting hypoxia with $PaO_2 < 8$ kPa despite maximal oxygen administration, progressive hypercapnia, severe acidosis (pH < 7.2), shock and depressed consciousness are indications for mechanical ventilation. Alveolar recruitment strategies using PEEP aid oxygenation and ventilator modes that avoid high peak pressures and alveolar hyperinflation are optimal. *Physiotherapy* and *bronchoscopy* may aid sputum clearance and sample collection for further microbiology. Steroids do not improve pneumonia resolution, but may be indicted (hydrocortisone 8 mg/h) in patients with septic shock who are poorly responsive to fluid and inotropic therapy.

Initial Antibiotic Therapy

Initial antibiotic therapy represents the 'best guess', according to pneumonia classification and likely organisms, as microbiological results are often not available for >24 h. Therapy is adjusted when results and antibiotic sensitivities are available. The American and British Thoracic Societies (ATS, BTS) recommendations for initial antibiotic therapy differ slightly and are as follows:

- **Non-hospitalised patients:** with less severe symptoms usually respond to oral monotherapy with amoxicillin 0.5–1 g tds (BTS), or a macrolide (e.g. clarithromycin 500 mg bd) (ATS/BTS) *or* doxycycline 100 mg od (ATS). Patients with severe symptoms or at risk for drug-resistant *S. pneumoniae* (e.g. recent antibiotics, comorbidity, alcoholism, immunosuppressive illness, recent travel to areas with high levels of *S. pneumoniae* resistance [e.g. Portugal, Spain]) are treated with a β-lactam (e.g. co-amoxiclav 625 mg tds) *plus* a macrolide or doxycycline; *or* an oral antipneumococcal fluoroquinolone alone (e.g. levofloxacin 500 mg od, moxifloxacin) (ATS).
- **Hospitalised patients:** antibiotic therapy must cover 'atypical' organisms and *S. pneumoniae* at admission. If not severe, the BTS suggests that combined ampicillin *plus* macrolide (oral or iv) may be adequate. In severe CAP, the BTS recommends intravenous therapy with co-amoxiclav

1.2 g tds *or* a second- or third-generation cephalosporin (e.g. cefuroxime 1.5 g tds iv) *plus* a macrolide (e.g. clarithromycin 500 mg bd). The ATS guidelines recommend intravenous therapy with a β-lactam (e.g. ceftriaxone 1–2 g od) *plus* an advanced macrolide (clarithromycin 500 mg bd) *or* an antipneumoccocal fluoroquinolone (e.g. levofloxacin 500 mg bd or moxafloxacin). Staphylococcal infection following influenza and *H. influenzae* in COPD should also be appropriately covered. An antipseudomonal agent may be required when there is underlying structural lung disease.

Hospital-Acquired (Nosocomial) Pneumonia

Hospital-acquired pneumonia (HAP) including *ventilator-associated pneumonia* (VAP) and *health-care associated pneumonia* (HCAP) affects 0.5–2% of hospitalised patients. Pathogenesis, causative organisms and outcome differ from community-acquired pneumonia (CAP). Preventative measures and early antibiotic therapy guided by awareness of the role of potential multidrug-resistant (MDR) pathogens improve outcome (Table 5.3). **Definitions:** for HAP, VAP and HCAP see Classification of Pneumonia.

Epidemiology

HAP is the second commonest nosocomial (hospital-acquired) infection in the USA (after wound infection) and the most important in terms of mortality. Available data suggest that it affects between 5 and 10 per 1,000 hospital admissions

TABLE 5.3. Risk factors for multidrug-resistant pathogens causing hospital-acquired pneumonia

- Antimicrobial therapy in the previous 90 days
- Current hospitalisation of >5 days
- High frequency of local antibiotic resistance
- Presence of risk factors for HCAP
  - Hospitalisation for >2 days in the previous 90 days
  - Residence in a nursing home
  - Home wound care or intravenous therapy
  - Chronic dialysis within 30 days
  - Family member with MDR pathogen
- Immunosuppressive disease and/or therapy

and lengthens hospital stay by 3–14 days/patient. Incidence is highest in surgical and ICU wards and in teaching hospitals. In ICU, HAP accounts for 25% of all infections and ~50% of prescribed antibiotics. The risk of HAP increases 6–20-fold during mechanical ventilation (MV) and occurs in 9–27% of intubated patients. VAP accounts for >80% of all HAPs. The risk of VAP is highest early in the course of hospital stay and is estimated to be 3%/day during the first 5 days of MV, 2%/day during days 5–10 of MV and 1%/day after this. As most MV is short term about 50% of all episodes of VAP occur during the first 4 days of MV.

Aetiology

HAP is caused by a wide spectrum of bacterial pathogens. Time of onset (i.e. early or late-onset HAP/VAP) and risk factors for infection with MDR organisms determine potential pathogens (Table 5.3). Aerobic Gram-negative bacilli (e.g. *Klebsiella pneumoniae, Pseudomonas aeruginosa, Escherichia coli, Acinetobacter* spp.) cause ~60–70% of infections and *Staphylococcus aureus* causes ~10–15%. *S. pneumoniae* and *H. influenzae* may be isolated in early onset HAP/VAP. In ICU, >50% *S. aureus* infections are methicillin-resistant (MRSA). In general, the bacteriology in non-ventilated and ventilated patients is similar. Pneumonia due to *S. aureus* is more common in

diabetics, head trauma and ICU patients. Reported rates of polymicrobial infections vary widely but are increasing and are especially high in patients with ARDS. Viral and fungal infections are rare in immunocompetent hosts.

Pathogenesis

Oropharyneal colonisation with enteric Gram-negative bacteria occurs in most hospitalised patients within a few days of admission due to immobility, impaired consciousness, instrumentation (e.g. nasogastric tubes, gastroscopy), inadequate attendant hygiene with cross infection or inhibition of gastric acid secretion (e.g. proton pump inhibitor therapy) (Figure 5.2). Subsequent aspiration of nasopharyngeal secretions (or gastric contents) due to supine positioning, reduced consciousness, difficulty swallowing, leakage past endotracheal-tube cuffs, infected biofilm in the endotracheal tube with subsequent embolisation to distal airways or direct inoculation of the airways during suctioning introduces these organisms into the LRT. Impaired mechanical, cellular and humoral host defences and inability to clear secretions (e.g. structural lung disease, sedation, MV, postoperative pain) promote ensuing infection. Haematogenous spread from distant infected sites (e.g. infected central lines) may also cause HAP.

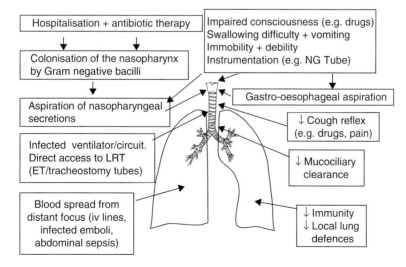

FIGURE 5.2. Pathogenesis of hospital-acquired pneumonia (HAP).

Risk Factors

Risk factors include those that predispose to CAP and factors associated with the development of MDR organisms and HAP pathogenesis (Tables 5.2 and 5.3, Figure 5.2). Critical risk factors include prolonged (>48 h) mechanical ventilation, duration of hospital or ICU stay, severity of illness (including APACHE score), presence of acute respiratory distress syndrome and medical comorbidity. In ventilated patients prior use of antibiotics appears protective, whereas continuous sedation, cardiopulmonary resuscitation, high ventilatory pressures, upper airway colonisation and duration of ventilation are independent risk factors. *Prevention*: Table 5.4 lists modifiable risk factors that reduce HAP incidence.

Diagnosis

Diagnosis of HAP is based on *both clinical and microbiological assessments* but may be difficult (especially in ventilated patients) as clinical features are often non-specific, patients may have concurrent illness (e.g. ARDS) and previous antibiotics limit microbiological evaluation. *Clinical criteria*: HAP is suspected if a patient develops new radiographic infiltrates (± hypoxaemia) with at least two of three clinical features suggestive of infection (e.g. temperature > 38°C, purulent sputum, leukocytosis or leukopaenia). Purulent tracheobronchitis may mimic many of the clinical features of HAP. *Diagnostic tests*: verify infection and determine the causative organism and antibiotic sensitivity. They include all the routine blood and radiographic tests used in CAP, blood cultures, CRP monitoring, diagnostic thoracocentesis of pleural effusions and LRT cultures including endotracheal aspirates and bronchioalveolar lavage in intubated patients. CT scanning aids diagnosis and detection of complications. *Complications:* are frequent with cavitation, abscesses, effusions and haemoptysis (Figure 5.3).

Management

Early diagnosis and treatment of HAP improves morbidity and mortality and requires constant vigilance in hospital patients. Antibiotic therapy must not be delayed while awaiting diagnostic tests and microbiological results.

TABLE 5.4. Risk factors for HAP and VAP

Unmodifiable risk factors	Modifiable risk factors
Host-related	*Host-related*
• Malnutrition	• Nutrition (e.g. enteral feeding)
• Age: >65, <5 years old	• Pain control, physiotherapy
• Diabetes	• Posture, kinetic beds
• Chronic disease (e.g. renal)	• Limit immunosuppressive
• Alcohol dependency	therapy
• Aspiration (e.g. epilepsy)	• Preoperative smoking
• Immunosuppression	cessation
(e.g. SLE)	
• Recent viral illness	*Therapy-related*
• Smoking	• Semi-recumbent position
• Obesity	(30° head up)
	• Early removal of iv lines, ET
Epidemiological factors	and NG tubes
• Environmental	• Avoid intubation +
(e.g. psitticosis)	re-intubation
• Occupational (e.g. Q fever)	• Minimise sedative use
• Travel abroad (e.g.	• Avoid gastric overdistention
paragonomiasis)	• Maintain ET cuff pressure
• Air conditioning	>20 cmH$_2$0
(e.g. Legionella)	• Subglottic aspiration during
	intubation
Therapy-related	• Drain and change ventilator
• Mechanical ventilation	circuits
• Postoperative	
	Infection control
	• Hand washing, sterile
	technique
	• Microbiological surveillance
	• Patient isolation

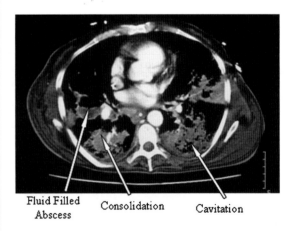

Fluid Filled Abscess   Consolidation   Cavitation

FIGURE 5.3. Computed tomography (CT) scan from a patient with hospital-acquired pneumonia showing consolidation, cavitation and abscess formation.

Supportive Therapy

Supportive therapy includes supplemental oxygen to maintain $PaO_2 > 8\,kPa$ (saturation > 90%) and intravenous fluids (± vasopressors or inotropes) to maintain a mean blood pressure >65 mmHg and urine output 0.5–1 mL/kg/min. *Ventilatory support* including non-invasive (e.g. CPAP, NIPPV) or mechanical ventilation may be required in respiratory failure (see CAP management). *Intensive insulin therapy* to maintain serum glucose levels between 4 and 6.5 mmol/L improves outcome. Vigorous *physiotherapy* and adequate *analgesia* aid sputum clearance postoperatively and in the immobilised patient. Avoid heavy sedation and paralytic agents that may depress cough. *Semi-recumbent nursing* of bed-bound patients with elevation of the bedhead to 30° reduces aspiration risk. *Continuous subglottic aspiration* using specially designed endotracheal tubes may reduce early onset VAP but frequency of ventilator circuit changes does not affect VAP incidence. *Stress ulcer prophylaxis* with either sucrulfate or proton pump inhibitors is acceptable although there is a trend to reduce VAP with sucrulfate. It is essential that modifiable risk factors are addressed (Table 5.4).

Antibiotic Therapy

Antibiotic therapy is empirical (as with CAP) while awaiting microbiological guidance. However, the causative organisms and suitable antibiotics differ from CAP. The initial key decisions are (i) whether the patient has risk factors for MDR organisms (Table 5.3), and (ii) whether the patient has early or late-onset HAP/VAP or HCAP, which determines the need for broad-spectrum (i.e. combination) antibiotic therapy. Figure 5.4 illustrates the recently published American Thoracic Society guidelines for initial, empiric antibiotic therapy. Initial therapy should be intravenous in all patients. About 50% of the initial, empiric treatment regimes will need modification due to either resistant organisms or failure to respond. However, it is important to try and get the antibiotic treatment 'right the first time' because mortality is lower in patients receiving effective initial antibiotic therapy compared to those that require a treatment change. Consequently, *local*

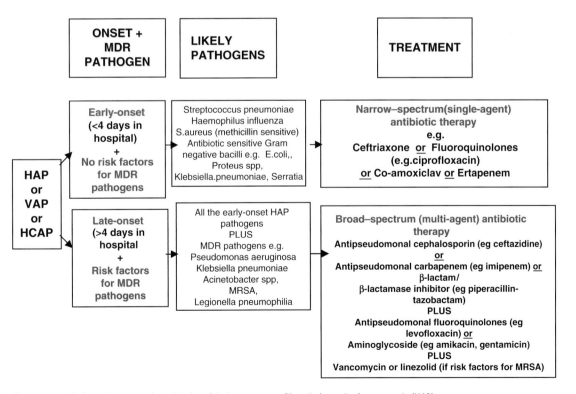

FIGURE 5.4. Likely pathogens and empirical antibiotic treatment of hospital-acquired pneumonia (HAP).

patterns of bacterial infection and antibiotic resistance should be used to establish the 'best empiric therapy regimen' for an individual hospital.

- In *early onset HAP/VAP* (<4 days in hospital) with no risk factors for MDR organisms, antibiotic *monotherapy* is advised with:

  ○ A β-lactam/β-lactamase inhibitor (e.g. piperacillin-tazobactam 4.5 g qds iv)
  ○ A third-generation cephalosporin (e.g. ceftazidime 2 g tds iv) or
  ○ A floroquinolone (e.g. ciprofloxacin 400 mg tds iv)

- In *late-onset HAP/VAP* (>4 days in hospital) or with risk factors for MDR pathogens (Table 5.4) and most HCAP *combination therapy*, with broad-spectrum antibiotics that cover MDR Gram-negative bacilli and MRSA, may be required. For example:

  ○ An antipseudomonal cephalosporin (e.g. ceftazidine 2 g tds iv), an antipseudomonal carbepenem (e.g. imipenem 0.5–1 g qds, meropenem 1 g tds iv), or a β-lactam/β-lactamase inhibitor (e.g. piperacillin-tazobactam 4.5 g qds iv).
  ○ *Plus* an antipseudomonal fluoroquinolone (e.g. ciprofloxacin 400 mg tds iv, levofloxacin 750 mg od iv) or aminoglycoside (e.g. gentamicin 7 mg/kg od iv, adjusted to maintain monitored trough levels <1 μg/mL).
  ○ *Plus* vancomycin 15 mg/kg bd (adjusted to maintain monitored trough levels 15–20 μg/mL) or linezolid 600 mg bd iv.
  ○ Adjunctive therapy with inhaled aerosolised aminoglycosides or polymyxin should be considered in patients not improving with systemic antibiotic therapy or who have VAP due to MDR Gram-negative pathogens and/or carbapenem-resistant *Acinetobacter* spp.

A short course of therapy (e.g. 7 days) is appropriate, if the clinical response is good. However, aggressive or resistant pathogens (e.g. *P. aeruginosa*, *S. Aureus*) may require treatment for 14–21 days, which improves subsequent survival. Overuse of antibiotics is avoided by tailoring antibiotic therapy to the results of lower respiratory tract cultures, withdrawing unnecessary antibiotics and shortening duration of therapy to the minimum effective period. Sterile cultures (in the absence of new antibiotics in the previous 72 h) virtually rules out the presence of HAP (94% negative predictive value for VAP) and withdrawal of antibiotic therapy should be considered. Although there is some evidence for a reduction in ICU-acquired HAP/VAP following prophylactic antibiotic administration, routine use is *not* recommended.

Mortality

The crude mortality rate for HAP may be as high as 30–70%, but many of these critically ill patients die of their underlying disease rather than pneumonia. The directly 'attributable mortality' due to HAP is estimated to be 33–50% in case-matched VAP studies. Delayed or ineffective antibiotic therapy, bacteraemia (especially with *P. aeruginosa* or *Acinetobacter* spp.), medical rather than surgical illness and VAP also increase mortality. *Early onset* HAP/VAP (defined as occurring within the first 4 days of hospitalisation) is usually caused by antibiotic-sensitive bacteria and carries a better prognosis than *late-onset* HAP/VAP (defined as occurring 5 days or more after hospitalisation), which is associated with MDR pathogens. However, in early onset HAP/VAP, prior antibiotic therapy or hospitalisation predisposes to MDR pathogens and is treated as late-onset HAP/VAP.

Other Pneumonias

Aspiration/Anaerobic Pneumonia

Bacteroides and other anaerobic infections follow aspiration of oropharyngeal contents due to impaired laryngeal competence (e.g. CVA) or reduced consciousness (e.g. drugs, alcohol) (Figure 5.5). Lung abscesses are common. Antibiotic therapy should include anaerobic coverage (e.g. metronidazole 500 mg tds iv). Large lung abscesses may require oral antibiotic therapy for several weeks.

Pneumonia During Immunosuppression

HIV, bone marrow transplant and chemotherapy patients are susceptible to viral (e.g. cytomegalovirus), fungal (e.g. aspergillus) and mycobacterial infections, in addition to the normal range of organisms. Severely immunocompromised patients require isolation, barrier nursing

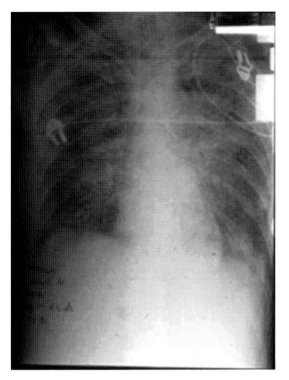

FIGURE 5.5. Aspiration pneumonia; chest x-ray (CXR) 6 h after aspiration of gastric contents.

and combined broad-spectrum antibiotic, antifungal (e.g. amphotericin) and antiviral (e.g. acyclovir) regimes. HIV patients with CD_4 counts $<200/mm^3$ are at high risk of opportunistic infections including *Pneumocystis carinii* pneumonia (PCP), toxoplasmosis and mycobacterium avian intracellulare. PCP is treated with steroids and high-dose co-trimoxazole.

Recurrent Pneumonia

Recurrent pneumonia with aerobic and anaerobic organisms occurs in cystic fibrosis and bronchiectasis. Pulmonary fibrosis with distorted architecture and frequent antibiotic usage result in MDR organisms and the need for broad-spectrum regimens adjusted according to microbiological results and antibiotic sensitivities.

Recommended Reading

1. BTS Guidelines for the management of community acquired pneumonia in adults. *Thorax.* 2001;56 (Suppl 4):1–68.
2. American Thoracic Society: Guidelines for the management of adults with community-acquired pneumonia; diagnosis, assessment of severity, microbial therapy and prevention. *Am J Respir Crit Care Med.* 2001;163:1730–1754.
3. BTS Guidelines for the management of community acquired pneumonia in adults – 2004 update. Accessed April 30, 2004. www.brit-thorack.org.uk
4. American Thoracic Society: Guidelines for the management of adults with hospital-acquired, ventilator-associated, and healthcare-associated pneumonia. *Am J Respir Crit Care Med.* 2005;171:388–416.
5. P. Tarsia, S. Aliberti, R. Cosentini, F. Blasi. Hospital-acquired pneumonia. *Breathe.* 2005;1:297–301.

6
Pleural Effusions in the Critically Ill

Philip S. Marino

Abstract Pleural effusions commonly occur in the critically ill and arise primarily through a combination of organ failure (cardiac, renal, hepatic), sepsis and poor nutrition leading to hypoalbuminaemia. The incidence varies considerably, with estimates ranging from 8% to 60% depending on whether clinical or radiological criteria are applied. Effusions are typically defined in terms of transudates (protein content <30 g/dL) and exudates (>30 g/dL). The nature and cause of a pleural effusion is usually determined by pleural fluid aspiration and analysis, together with non-invasive imaging such as chest radiography, ultrasound and computerised tomography (CT). Management is dependent on the underlying cause (e.g. heart failure, pneumonia), effusion size and symptom severity. Treatment may be initially medical (thoracocentesis, diuretics, antibiotics), though surgical intervention (intercostal drains, pleurodesis, pleural shunts) may be required in more complex cases such as empyema or neoplasia.

Introduction

Pleural effusions are a common medical problem, particularly in the critically ill, occurring in 8–10% of ICU patients based on clinical and radiological findings, though an effusion may be detected in up to 60% of patients with ultrasonography.[1–3] A pleural effusion represents the accumulation of fluid in the pleural space and may be caused by a wide variety of disorders (see Pleural Fluid Analysis and Imaging). The nature of the effusion depends on the underlying cause, but several factors may contribute to their development in the critically ill such as sepsis, organ failure (cardiac, renal, hepatic), hypoalbuminaemia and large volume intravenous fluid resuscitation.[1] This chapter will review the pathophysiology, aetiology, investigation and management of pleural effusions.

Patho-Physiology

The pleura are comprised of five main structures[4] (Figure 6.1). The outermost layer is formed by extra-pleural tissue, consisting of branches of the intercostal and internal mammary arteries, lymphatic vessels and extra-pleural interstitium. Beneath this layer lie the parietal and visceral pleurae, each comprising a layer of mesothelial cells separated by the pleural space or cavity. The innermost layer is formed by the lung edge comprising of alveoli, interstitial fluid, blood and lymphatic vessels.

In health the pleural cavity contains 1 mL of fluid producing a fine film between the parietal and visceral pleura. Pleural fluid is normally formed through filtration of fluid from blood vessels in the extra-pleural tissues via the parietal pleura along a pressure gradient into the pleural cavity. Fluid then drains out of the pleural cavity via lymphatics in the parietal pleura which eventually drain into the mediastinal lymph nodes.

This balance may be disrupted through several mechanisms resulting in fluid accumulation within the pleural space. For example, a transudate will form when pulmonary capillary pressure is raised

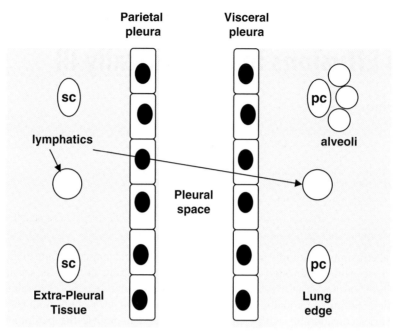

FIGURE 6.1.　Pleural anatomy.

(e.g. left ventricular failure, renal failure) or oncotic pressure is reduced (e.g. hypo-albuminaemia). Exudates predominantly occur when the permeability of the pleural membrane is increased by infection, inflammatory disease or malignancy. Alternatively, obstruction of lymphatic flow by malignancy may also result in an exudative pleural effusion.

Types of Pleural Effusion

Pleural effusions can be categorised according to aetiology, biochemical composition and macroscopic appearance leading to four main types being described:

- Transudates
- Exudates
- Haemothorax
- Chylous effusion (chylothorax/pseudochylothorax)

Transudates

The term transudate refers to any effusion with a protein content <30 g/dL in the presence of a normal serum albumin.[5] Transudates usually develop through a relative imbalance between pulmonary capillary pressure and plasma oncotic pressure. The most common causes of transudates are left ventricular failure, liver cirrhosis, renal failure and protein losing enteropathy; however, a wide variety of other conditions may also be implicated as outlined in Table 6.1.

Exudates

Exudates often develop in response to infection and/or inflammation adjacent to or within the pleural cavity. The protein content is raised (≥30 g/dL) relative to the serum protein level and an inflammatory cell infiltrate is frequently present.[5] Exudates are most commonly associated with pneumonia, neoplasia, connective tissue disorders and pulmonary infarction. A comprehensive list of causes is given in Table 6.1.

Haemothorax

A haemothorax is often diagnosed by the presence of frank blood within the pleural fluid.

TABLE 6.1. Aetiology of transudates and exudates

Transudate	Exudate
• Left ventricular failure	• Pneumonia (bacterial, fungal, TB)
• Cirrhosis	• Neoplasia
• Hypoalbuminaemia	• Pulmonary infarction
• Nephrotic syndrome	• Rheumatoid arthritis
• Peritoneal dialysis	• Pancreatic disease (pancreatitis,
• Protein losing	pseudocyst)
enteropathy	• Collagen vascular disease
• Hypothyroidism	(Wegener's granulomatosis, SLE,
• Pulmonary embolus	Churg–Strauss)
• Constrictive pericarditis	• Benign asbestos-related pleural
• Superior vena cava	disease
obstruction	• Dressler's syndrome
• Urinothorax	• Intra-abdominal abscess
• Meig's syndrome	(subphrenic, hepatic, splenic)
	• Oesophageal rupture
	• Drug-induced (e.g. amiodarone)
	• Radiotherapy
	• Yellow-nail syndrome

However, if the fluid is only blood-stained, a diagnosis can only be established by measuring the pleural fluid haematocrit. A haemothorax is present if the pleural fluid haematocrit is more than half of the patient's peripheral blood haematocrit. The condition is associated with malignancy, trauma (including pneumothorax), post-cardiac injury syndrome and benign asbestos pleural disease.[6] Other causes include large pulmonary embolism with infarction, aortic dissection and coagulopathy.

Chylous Effusion

A chylothorax refers to the accumulation of lymph (or chyle) within the pleural cavity, with the fluid appearing milk-like in nature, resulting from the disruption of the thoracic duct or its tributary vessels.[7] The most common causes for a chylothorax are neoplasia (~50%; particularly lymphoma), infection (tuberculosis), trauma and surgery (25%; predominantly neck and chest). A pseudochylothorax results from the progressive accumulation of cholesterol crystals in a chronic pleural effusion, with progressively thickened and fibrotic pleura. This phenomenon is usually associated with chronic rheumatoid pleurisy, tuberculosis and inadequately treated empyema, though it may occur with artificial pneumothoraces.

Investigations

Pleural Fluid Analysis

Direct sampling of pleural fluid is essential in the diagnosis and treatment of pleural effusions. Various parameters have been studied though only a few have been shown to aid diagnosis.[6] The following variables should be measured in all cases:

- Protein
- Lactate dehydrogenase (LDH)
- pH
- Glucose
- Microscopy, culture and sensitivity
- Cytology
- Amylase
- Other—lipids (cholesterol, triglycerides), alanine deaminase (ADA)

Protein and LDH

The protein content of pleural fluid has conventionally been used to discriminate between transudates and exudates with a protein level of less than 30 g/dL and greater than 30 g/dL, respectively.[5] These values depend on the serum protein being normal which is frequently not the case in the critically ill. In addition, both pleural and serum protein concentration may be altered by diuretic therapy which is often administered in the ICU.

In view of these limitations, Light's criteria were developed to differentiate exudates from transudates using pleural protein and LDH measurements.[5] An exudate is present if one or more of the following criteria are fulfilled:

- Pleural fluid/serum protein ratio >0.5
- Pleural fluid/serum LDH ratio >0.6
- Pleural fluid LDH >2/3 the upper limit of normal serum LDH

The sensitivity and specificity of these criteria are 81% and 91% respectively, and Light's criteria have been widely adopted as the most accurate method for differentiating exudates from transudates.

pH and Glucose

Pleural fluid pH has been used as a marker of infection or inflammation within the pleural cavity. A pH level of <7.2 (with normal blood pH) is highly indicative of pleural infection, though similar values may occur with malignancy, collagen vascular disease (e.g. rheumatoid arthritis, SLE) and oesophageal rupture.[8] These conditions are also associated with low pleural glucose level (<3 mmol), with readings below 2 mmol present in pleural sepsis and rheumatoid arthritis.[9]

Microscopy, Culture and Sensitivity

Differential white cell analysis may help to characterise and diagnose the cause of a pleural effusion by identifying a predominant cell type. For example, polymorph (neutrophil)-rich effusions are often seen in cases of pneumonia, pulmonary embolism, viral infection, acute tuberculosis or benign asbestos-related pleural disease.[6] Lymphocytic effusions are typically found in tuberculosis, neoplasia (especially lymphoma), sarcoidosis, rheumatoid arthritis and chylothoraces. An eosinophilic effusion (>10% cell count) may arise in pneumonia but can also occur in neoplasia, tuberculosis, pulmonary infarction, Churg–Strauss, benign asbestos-related pleural disease, parasitic disease and idiosyncratic drug reaction.

All specimens should be sent for routine culture and sensitivity with additional samples required for TB and/or fungal culture if there is a high index of suspicion (e.g. immunocompromised or patients from endemic areas).

Cytology

Neoplasia may be diagnosed in up to 60% of cases from pleural fluid aspirates alone.[10] Diagnostic yield can be improved by repeated sampling, so further aspiration should be considered if malignancy is strongly suspected.

Amylase

Pleural amylase is raised in specific conditions, aiding diagnosis in certain circumstances. Elevated amylase levels (pleural/serum ratio >1) are observed in acute pancreatitis, pancreatic pseudocyst, oesophageal rupture, pleural malignancy and ruptured ectopic pregnancy.[11] Measurement of pancreatic and salivary isoenzymes may help to differentiate oesophageal rupture from pancreatic disease.

Lipid Profile

Chylothoraces and pseudochylothoraces can be distinguished from one another by lipid analysis of the pleural fluid.[12] A chylothorax will usually have a raised triglyceride level, typically >1.24 mmol/L, with chylomicrons present but no cholesterol crystals. A chylous effusion can normally be excluded if the triglyceride is <0.56 mmol/L. In a pseudochylous effusion the triglyceride level is low but the cholesterol level is raised (>5.18 mmol/L), with cholesterol crystals often present on microscopy. An empyema may occasionally appear similar to a chylous effusion but can be distinguished by centrifugation which leaves a clear supernatant and cellular sediment on separation.

Adenosine Deaminase (ADA)

Raised ADA levels have been found in pleural fluid aspirates from patients with tuberculosis.[13] However, ADA may also be elevated in pleural sepsis, neoplasia and certain connective tissue disorders, so it must be interpreted in the context of each clinical case.

Imaging

Chest Radiograph

Most pleural effusions in the critically ill are identified following a routine chest radiograph (Figure 6.2a). An effusion is usually visible when 200 mL or more of fluid is present, though smaller effusions (50 mL) may be detected on lateral films by loss of the posterior costophrenic angle.[14] Ventilated patients are often imaged supine causing loss of the fluid layer, though other radiological features remain that still allow diagnosis (Figure 6.2b). There may be hazy opacification of the hemithorax with preservation of the vascular structures. Poor delineation of the ipsilateral hemidiaphragm and thickening of the minor fissure may also be present.

Occasionally, sub-pulmonic effusions will occur and can be difficult to identify on routine chest radiographs. Subtle features may include elevation of the hemi-diaphragm with lateral peaking and downward sloping of the major fissure. However, the chest radiograph frequently underestimates

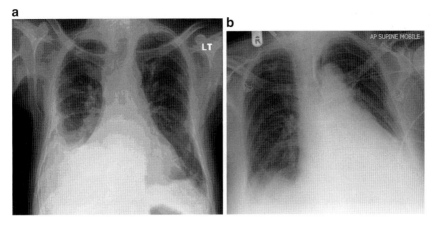

FIGURE 6.2. Typical CXRs of (**a**) a right-sided pleural effusion and (**b**) bilateral pleural effusions in a supine patient.

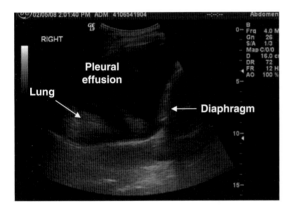

FIGURE 6.3. Ultrasound appearance of a pleural effusion.

the nature and size of a pleural effusion so that other imaging modalities such as ultrasound or computerised tomography (CT) are required.

Ultrasound

Ultrasonography allows more accurate assessment of the nature, size and site of pleural collections than conventional chest radiography[15,16] (Figure 6.3). The superior resolution can show fibrinous septation, loculation and distinguish pleural thickening from fluid. Exudates are invariably septated and homogenously echogenic (particularly in infection or haemorrhage). Ultrasound is frequently used to guide thoracocentesis, particularly in loculated effusions or when previous pleural aspiration has failed, with success rates of up to 97%.[17] Complication rates are also reduced with some studies reporting low rates of pneumothorax

(1.3%) in mechanically ventilated patients.[18,19] Its principle advantage is mobility, allowing repeatable, detailed imaging at the bedside.

Computerised Tomography (CT)

CT scanning with contrast enhancement provides high-resolution images of the pleura and underlying lung parenchyma (Figure 6.4a). Pleural disease may be distinguished from parenchymal lung pathology (e.g. pneumonia or neoplasia) and CT can help to differentiate benign from malignant pleural disease. The main features of malignant pleural disease include nodular and/or circumferential pleural thickening, particularly involving the mediastinal and parietal pleura.[20] CT scanning should be performed prior to pleural drainage to provide better anatomical definition.

The presence, nature and severity of pleural infection may also be assessed by contrast-enhanced CT (Figure 6.4b). Empyemas usually appear lenticular in shape with compression of the adjacent lung parenchyma, whilst lung abscesses may have poorly defined margins.[21] CT pulmonary angiogram should be considered in patients with a persistent, undiagnosed pleural effusion despite extensive investigation.[6]

Diagnostic Procedures

Bronchoscopy

Fibre-optic bronchoscopy has a limited role in the investigation of pleural effusion. It may aid

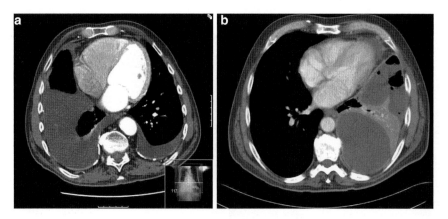

FIGURE 6.4. Typical CT appearance of (**a**) a pleural effusion and (**b**) an empyema with loculations and pleural thickening.

diagnosis in cases where an underlying malignancy is suspected (e.g. haemoptysis, chronic cough, weight loss) or there is associated consolidation/collapse indicative of possible bronchial obstruction by tumour or a foreign body.[6] This should ideally be performed after pleural drainage to avoid distortion of the lung anatomy due to airway compression by the effusion.

Pleural Biopsy

Percutaneous biopsy is normally undertaken when pleural malignancy or tuberculosis is suspected, particularly in patients with a chronic pleural effusion in whom all previous investigations have failed to yield a diagnosis.[6] The procedure can be performed blind with an Abram's needle, at the same time as pleural aspiration, or under image guidance with contrast-enhanced CT using a true-cut biopsy needle.

Previous studies have shown blind biopsy to yield a diagnosis in an extra 7–27% of cases following thoracocentesis, with total diagnostic rates of 57% and 75% for carcinoma and tuberculosis.[22–24] However, the diagnostic rates for both conditions increases further when pleural biopsy is performed under image guidance. The diagnostic yield for pulmonary tuberculosis increases to 80–90% when undertaken in conjunction with pleural fluid analysis and Ziehl–Nielson staining for acid-alcohol fast bacilli (AAFB) and culture for tuberculosis.[25,26] The most common complications are pneumothorax (3–15%), haemothorax (<2%), site bleeding (<1%) and fever (<1%).[25]

Thoracoscopy

Video-assisted thoracoscopy allows direct visualisation of the pleural space, considerably improving diagnosis by draining all the pleural fluid for analysis, permitting inspection of the pleura and thereby facilitating pleural biopsy. The technique is normally reserved for those individuals with a chronic pleural effusion in whom all other investigations have failed to provide a diagnosis.

The procedure may be performed under local anaesthesia, so-called medical thoracoscopy, allowing non-ventilated patients with significant co-morbidities who cannot tolerate general anaesthesia, such as the elderly, to be investigated. Ventilated patients may receive surgical intervention during thoracoscopy (e.g. decortication, pleurodesis) under general anaesthesia. Serious complications such as major haemorrhage are rare but surgical emphysema (6.9%) and cardiac arrythmias (0.35%) have been reported in previous case series.[27]

Management

Several factors must be considered when determining the treatment of a pleural effusion. These include the underlying cause, size, chronicity, patient age and co-morbidities. In addition to establishing the diagnosis, the main steps in management are treatment of the underlying cause, drainage and preventative measures should recurrence occur.

Treatment of the Underlying Cause

Attempts should be made to treat the underlying condition in all cases in order to aid recovery and prevent recurrence. In certain situations this may be sufficient to achieve resolution of the effusion, for example, diuretics in left ventricular failure.

Left Ventricular Failure

Pleural effusions of varying size occur in up to 80% of patients with cardiac failure. The majority of cases will normally resolve with optimisation of medical therapy. Patients should receive appropriate diuretic therapy with an angiotensin converting enzyme (ACE) inhibitor or angiotensin II receptor antagonist and a β-blocker introduced once tolerable. Spironolactone may be started in those patients with more severe cardiac failure (NYHA grade 3 or 4). However, large effusions causing significant symptoms or respiratory compromise (difficulty with mechanical ventilation or weaning) may not resolve rapidly with medical therapy, and will still require either thoracocentesis or chest drain insertion.

Pneumonia and Empyema

All patients with empyema or complicated parapneumonic effusion should receive antibiotic therapy in addition to having intercostal drain insertion. The type of antibiotic regimen used depends on the whether the infection is hospital or community acquired, local bacterial prevalence and antibiotic policy. Ideally, antibiotic therapy should be guided by pleural fluid culture and sensitivities.

The organisms most commonly associated with community-acquired infection are *Streptococcus pneumoniae*, *Haemophilus influenzae* and *Staphylococcus aureus*.[28] The British Thoracic Society (BTS) guidelines on the management of pleural infection advise that intravenous empirical therapy should consist of either a second-generation cephalosporin (e.g. cefuroxime) with metronidazole or a penicillin with a quinolone (e.g. benzyl penicillin and ciprofloxacin). Meropenem and metronidazole or clindamycin, with or without a cephalosporin, may be used in those individuals with penicillin allergy. Aminoglycosides do not adequately penetrate the pleural cavity and are generally avoided. There is no data regarding duration of therapy, though treatment for 3 weeks is usually advocated.[29] Patients may be converted to an oral regimen if a prolonged course of treatment is recommended, and the BTS guidelines advise using a beta-lactamase-inhibiting penicillin (e.g. co-amoxiclav), with or without metronidazole, or clindamycin alone.

Pleural infection can also occur with atypical bacteria, although significant disease is rare.[30,31] Small effusions are seen in 5–20% of patients with mycoplasma pneumoniae, and are usually reactive in nature. Similarly, effusions associated with legionella pneumonia tend to be insignificant and self-resolving. Treatment with a macrolide antibiotic is recommended for effusions associated with atypical bacterial infection.

Hospital-acquired pleural infection usually occurs in conjunction with nosocomial pneumonia or chest trauma/surgery. Infection may be due to aerobes, both Gram positive and negative, and/or anaerobes. Empirical therapy must cover this broad spectrum of organisms with specific activity against pseudomonas and staphylococcus. The BTS guidelines advise using piperacillin-tazobactam, meropenem or a third-generation cephalosporin such as ceftazidime.[29] Mixed infection with *Streptococcus milleri* and anaerobes has been documented and is associated with significant mortality.[32] In these circumstances clindamycin, with or without a cephalosporin, may be considered.

Neoplasia

The majority of malignant pleural effusions require chest drain insertion or surgical intervention. In a small proportion the effusion will resolve after treatment of the underlying malignancy with chemotherapy, an example being small cell carcinoma of the lung, which is normally highly chemosensitive. However, chemotherapy may not be feasible in the critically ill patient with significant co-morbidities, particularly in the presence of severe sepsis.

Connective Tissue Disease

Disease modifying therapies such as corticosteroids and immunosuppressant drugs may need to be initiated in those with active disease in addition to performing pleural drainage. The opportunity to introduce these agents may again be limited by the patient's co-morbidities.

Thoracocentesis

Drainage of pleural effusions improves ventilation and cardio-pulmonary haemodynamics, shortens duration of mechanical ventilation and reduces ICU length of stay.[33] Therapeutic thoracocentesis is normally performed under local anaesthesia by inserting a suitably sized cannula (16 or 18 gauge) attached to a three-way tap and 50 mL luer lock syringe.[6] It is best practice to identify the point of drainage using ultrasonography. The procedure is most suitable for patients with small- to moderate-sized effusions (<500 mL), though up to 1 L may be aspirated, and offers certain advantages over conventional chest drain insertion. It is minimally invasive, and carries a lower risk of complications such as pneumothorax, especially when performed under ultrasound guidance. Thoracocentesis also tends to be better tolerated than drain insertion, particularly in patients with advanced cardiorespiratory disease who may require non-invasive ventilation. However, it has the disadvantage of being time-consuming, particularly for large effusions, and repeated intervention may be required in the event of recurrence. It is not suitable in patients with pleural sepsis.

Intercostal Chest Drain

Percutaneous chest drain insertion is regarded as the definitive form of treatment in the majority of cases. It is indicated in patients with moderate to large pleural effusions, often loculated, particularly when there is evidence of respiratory compromise (e.g. difficulty with ventilation or weaning) or confirmed pleural sepsis (empyema or complicated para-pneumonic effusion).[6,29]

Traditionally, large bore chest drains (size > or = 24) have been used to ensure adequate pleural drainage, but recently there has been a trend towards using small bore (size 10–14) Seldinger chest drains. They are considered to be less invasive, easier to insert and therefore better tolerated.[34,35] Small-scale studies have shown no significant difference in successful pleural drainage between large and small bore drains. However,

these were not randomised, controlled studies and did not assess the effect on the length of stay, duration of mechanical ventilation or hospital mortality. At present, large bore chest drains should be reserved for patients with empyema and large loculated pleural effusions. If smaller Seldinger drains are inserted blockage should be prevented by regular flushing with normal saline (25–50 mL aliquots) 2–4 times a day.[6]

Chest drains may occlude or fail to drain the effusion adequately, particularly when the effusion is loculated or purulent. If minimal or no fluid is obtained, a repeat chest radiograph should be performed in the first instance, to check that the drain is correctly placed, and to establish whether or not a collection remains. Occasionally, the chest radiograph is inconclusive and further imaging with CT is required.[6] If the drain is kinked or displaced it should be re-positioned, and if blocked an attempt should be made to flush it with 25–50 mL of normal saline. A new drain should be inserted and the original removed if it remains blocked. Suction may be applied at low pressure (10 cmH$_2$O or less) if the drain output remains problematic or resolution is slow.[36]

Until recently, fibrinolytic agents such as intrapleural streptokinase were used to aid drainage of loculated effusions, but a recent randomised controlled trial has shown no significant benefit in terms of resolution, length of hospital stay or mortality.[37] Clinical trials with alternative intrapleural agents such as DNAse are currently in progress.

Pleurodesis

This is normally performed in patients with recurrent pleural effusions, particularly those with malignant disease, to prevent further fluid accumulation. Pleurodesis involves the instillation of a sclerosing agent into the pleural cavity to induce a diffuse, inflammatory response followed by an intense fibrotic reaction causing adhesion between the visceral and parietal pleurae.

A number of agents have been used to achieve chemical pleurodesis, with varying degrees of success. In the past, tetracycline and bleomycin were used (doses 1–1.5 g and 60 units, respectively) with reported success rates of 50–90%.[38–41] These agents have now been superseded by sterile talc, due to its greater clinical effectiveness with response rates of 80–100% in published case series.[39,41,42] The talc (normally 5 g) may be inserted via a chest drain as a suspension or 'slurry', or instilled at thoracoscopy using an atomiser (so-called 'talc poudrage'). Similar success rates have been reported for both techniques.

The sclerosant may be instilled via the chest drain in the ICU or pleurodesis may be performed using video-assisted thorascopy in theatre. The latter approach allows the sclerosing agent to be instilled under direct visualisation increasing the effectiveness of the procedure. Once the sclerosant is inserted, the chest drain is normally clamped for 1 h and the patient rotated (if possible), though no evidence currently exists to support this approach. The chest drain is usually removed when the amount of fluid draining is less than 150 mL/day.[43] Patients may experience fever, pleuritic chest pain and nausea after pleurodesis, but serious side effects (e.g. empyema, acute lung injury, pneumonitis) are rare. Pain can be reduced by pre-medication with an opiate, with or without an anxiolytic (preferably a benzodiazepine), and inserting lignocaine (3 mg/kg; up to 250 mg maximum) prior to administering the sclerosant.[44] Caution must be exercised in those patients with significant cardiac disease.

Pleurodesis may fail in certain circumstances, the most common reason being excessive fluid within the pleural cavity (drainage still>250 mL/day). Although the procedure can be repeated using an alternative sclerosant, if that is also unsuccessful further attempts are likely to be futile and the drain may be removed. In some cases, the lung may not re-expand following drain insertion, due to the development of a fibrothorax trapping the underlying lung and preventing contact between the visceral and parietal pleura. In both of these situations, surgical intervention may be required to allow lung re-expansion and successful pleurodesis.

Surgery

Surgical intervention should be considered when pleural sepsis persists, and in patients with malignant or chronic pleural effusions that have not resolved with medical therapy (i.e. antibiotics, chest drain insertion). No specific criteria exist regarding referral for surgery, and the nature of the procedure performed will depend on various factors including the patient's underlying pathology, age, co-morbidities and the surgical facilities available. A surgical opinion should be sought when pleural infection persists beyond 7 days, with the aim of removing any residual infected fluid/tissue and preventing fibrothorax formation.[45] The procedures undertaken most frequently are video-assisted thoracoscopic surgery (VATS), open thoracic drainage and thoracotomy with decortication. VATS has become increasingly favoured in the treatment of chronic pleural effusions and pleural sepsis. The procedure requires double lumen intubation under general anaesthesia and has the specific advantage of allowing direct visualisation of the pleura facilitating decortication, biopsy, pleurodesis and chest drain placement.

VATS may not be possible in certain patients, particularly those with malignant disease, when pleurodesis has failed or a trapped lung has developed. Long-term indwelling pleural catheters and pleuroperitoneal shunts may be inserted in this situation under thoracoscopic guidance or by mini-thoracotomy. Long-term tunnelled pleural catheter insertion has been shown to be more effective than chemical pleurodesis via a chest drain in terms of length of hospital stay, quality of life, symptom scores, spontaneous pleurodesis and failure rates.[46] Pleuroperitoneal shunts consist of a valved chamber (containing two unidirectional valves) with pleural and peritoneal fenestrated catheters at either end. The device is pressure activated and needs regular manual compression. Shunt insertion is usually well tolerated with low post-operative morbidity and mortality rates.[47] The most common complications are localised infection (up to 14%), shunt occlusion (12–25%) and seeding of the pleural tract by tumour.

In non-ventilated patients who are unfit for general anaesthesia, further chest drain insertion under image guidance may be considered for loculated collections. Alternatively, surgical rib resection and open drainage may be performed under local anaesthesia.[6]

Nutritional Support

Poor nutrition and hypoalbuminaemia have both been shown to increase mortality in patients with pleural infection.[48] They are thought to cause immunodeficiency leading to delayed recovery. Nutritional support should therefore be initiated as soon as possible.

Summary

Pleural effusions are common in the critically ill. There are many different causes and management is dependent on establishing the type and size of the effusion. Management should focus on diagnosis, treatment of the underlying cause, drainage, prevention and general supportive measures.

References

1. Azoulay E. Pleural effusions in the intensive care unit. *Curr Opin Pulm Med.* 2003;9(4): 291–297.
2. Mattison LE, Coppage L, Alderman DF, Herlong JO, Sahn SA.. Pleural effusions in the medical ICU: prevalence, causes and clinical implications. *Chest.* 1997;111(4): 1018–1023.
3. Fartoukh M, Azoulay E, Galliot, et al. Clinically documented pleural effusions in medical ICU patients: how useful is routine thoracocentesis? *Chest.* 2002;121(1): 178–184.
4. Antunes G, Neville E, Duffy J, Ali N. On behalf of BTS Pleural Disease Group. BTS guidelines for the management of malignant pleural effusions. *Thorax.* 2003;58(Suppl II):ii29–ii38.
5. Light RW, Macgregor MI, Luchsinger PC, Ball, WC Jr. Pleural effusions: the diagnostic separation of transudates and exudates. *Ann Intern Med.* 1972;77:507–513.
6. Maskell NA, Butland RJA. On behalf of BTS Pleural Disease Group. BTS guidelines for the investigation of a unilateral pleural effusion in adults. *Thorax.* 2003;58(Suppl II): ii8–ii17.
7. Hillerdal G. Chylothorax and pseudochylothorax. *Eur Resp J.* 1997;10:1150–1156.
8. Good JT Jr, Taryle DA, Maulitz RM, Kaplan RL, Sahn SA. The diagnostic value of pleural fluid pH. *Chest.* 1980;78:55–59.
9. Light RW, Ball WCJ. Glucose and amylase in pleural effusions. *JAMA.* 1973;225:257–259.
10. Garcia L. The value of multiple fluid specimens in the cytological diagnosis of malignancy. *Mod Pathol.* 1994;7:665–668.
11. Sahn SA. The pleura. *Am Rev Resp Dis.* 1988;138: 184–234.
12. Hillerdal G. Chylothorax and pseudochylothorax. *Eur Respir J.* 1997;10:1150–1156.
13. Burgess LJ, Maritz FJ, Le Roux I, Taljaard JJ. Use of adenosine deaminase as a diagnostic tool for tuberculous pleurisy. *Thorax.* 1995;50:672–674.
14. Blackmore CC, Black WC, Dallas RV, Crow HC. Pleural fluid volume estimation: a chest radiograph prediction rule. *Acad Radiol.* 1996;3:103–109.
15. Vignan P, Chastagner C, Berkane V, et al. Quantitative assessment of pleural effusions in the critically ill patients by means of ultrasonography. *Crit Care Med.* 2005;33(8):1757–1763.
16. Balik M, Plasil P, Waldauf P, et al. Ultrasound estimation of volume of pleural fluid in mechanically ventilated patients. *Intensive Care Med.* 2006;32(2): 318–321.
17. O'Moore PV, Mueller PR, Simeone JF, et al. Sonographic guidance in diagnostic and therapeutic interventions in the pleural space. *AJR.* 1987;149: 103–109.
18. Mayo PH, Goltz HL, Tafredi M, Doelkam P. Safety of ultrasound guided thoracocentesis in patients on mechanical ventilation. *Chest.* 2004;125(3):1059–1062.
19. Mynarek G, Brabrand K, Jakobsen JA, Kolbenstvedt A. Complication following ultrasound guided thoracocentesis. *Acta Radiol.* 2004;45(5):519–522.
20. Leung AN, Muller NL, Miller RR. CT in differential diagnosis of diffuse pleural disease. *AJR.* 1990; 154:3–92.
21. Muller NL. Imaging of the pleura. *Radiology.* 1993;186:297–309.
22. Nance KV, Shermer RW, Askin FB. Diagnostic efficacy of pleural biopsy as compared with that of pleural fluid examination. *Mod Pathol.* 1991;4:320–324.
23. Prakash UB, Reiman HM. Comparison of needle biopsy with cytologic analysis for the evaluation of pleural effusion: analysis of 414 cases. *Mayo Clin Proc.* 1985;60:158–164.
24. Tomlinson JR. Invasive procedures in the diagnosis of pleural disease. *Semin Respir Med.* 1987; 9:30–36.
25. Poe RH, Israel RH, Utell MJ, Hall WJ, Greenblatt DW, Kallay MC. Sensitivity, specificity and predictive values of closed pleural biopsy. *Arch Intern Med.* 1984;144:325–328.
26. Escudero BC, Garcia CM, Cuesta CB, et al. Cytologic and bacteriologic analysis analysis of fluid and pleural biopsy specimens with Cope's needle. Study of 414 patients. *Arch Intern Med.* 1990;150:1190–1194.
27. Viskum K, Erik B. Complications of thoracoscopy. *Poumon Coeur.* 1981;37:25–28.
28. Huchon G, Woodhead M. Guidelines for management of adult community-acquired pneumonia lower respiratory tract infections. European study on Community-acquired Pneumonia (ESOCAP) Committee. *Eur Respir J.* 1998;11:986–991.

29. Maskell NA, Butland RJA. On behalf of BTS Pleural Disease Group. BTS guidelines for the management of pleural infection. *Thorax*. 2003;58(Suppl II) : ii18–ii28.

30. Kroboth FJ (1983) Clinicoradiographic correlation with extent of Legionnaires' disease. *AJR*. 1983;141: 263–268.

31. Mansel JK, Rosenow ECI, Smith TF, Martin JW Jr. Mycoplasma pneumoniae pneumonia. *Chest*. 1989;95:639–646.

32. Shinzato T, Saito A. The *Streptococcus milleri* group as a cause of pulmonary infections. *Clin Infect Dis*. 1995;21(Suppl 3):S328–S343

33. Ahmed SH, Ouzounian SP, Dirusso S, Sullivan T, Savino J, Del Guercio, L. Hemodynamic and pulmonary changes after drainage of significant pleural effusions in critically ill, mechanically ventilated surgical patients. *J Trauma*. 2004;57(6):1184–1188.

34. Silverman SG, Mueller PR, Saini S, et al. Thoracic empyema: management with image-guided catheter drainage. *Radiology*. 1988;169:5–9.

35. Ulmer JL, Choplin RH, Reed JC. Image-guided catheter drainage of the infected pleural space. *J Thorac Imaging*. 1991;6:65–73.

36. Munnell ER Thoracic drainage. *Ann Thorac Surg*. 1997;63:1497–1502.

37. Maskell NA, Davies CW, Ninm AJ, et al. First multicenter intrapleural sepsis trial (MIST1) Group. UK controlled trial of intrapleural streptokinase for pleural infection. *N Eng J Med*. 2005;352(9): 865–874.

38. Martinez-Moragon E, Aparicio J, Rogada MC, Sanchis J, Sanchis F, Gil-Suay V. Pleurodesis in malignant pleural effusions: a randomised study of tetracycline versus bleomycin. *Eur Respir J*. 1997;10: 2380–2383.

39. Zimmer PW, Hill M, Casey K, Harvey, Low DE. Prospective randomised trial slurry vs bleomycin in pleurodesis for symptomatic malignant pleural effusions. *Chest*. 1997;112:430–434.

40. Hartman DL, Gaither JM, Kesler KA, Mylet DM, Brown JW, Mathur PN. Comparison of insufflated talc under thoracoscopic guidance with standard tetracycline and bleomycin pleurodesis for control of malignant pleural effusions. *J Thorac Cardiovasc Surg*. 1993;105:743–747.

41. Tan C, Sedrakyan A, Browne J, Swift S, Treane T. The evidence on the effectiveness of management for malignant pleural effusions: a systematic review. *Eur J Cardiothoracic Surg*. 2006;29(5):829–838.

42. Weissberg D, Ben-Zeev I. Talc pleurodesis. Experience with 360 patients (1993). *J Thorac Cardovasc Surg*. 1993;106:689–695.

43. Sahn SA. Pleural disease related to metastatic malignancies. *Eur Respir J*. 1997;10:1907–913.

44. Wooten SA, Barbarash RA, Strange CL, Sahn SA. Systemic absorption of tetracycline and lidocaine following intrapleural instillation. Chest. 1998;94: 960–963.

45. Pathula V, Krellenstein DJ. Early aggressive surgical management of parapneumonic empyemas. *Chest*. 1994;105:832–836.

46. Tremblay A, Michoud G. Single center experience with 250 tunnelled pleural catheter insertion for malignant pleural effusion. Chest. 2006;192(2): 362–368.

47. Genc O, Petrou M, Laddas G, Goldstraw P. The long term morbidity of pleuro-peritoneal shunts in the management of recurrent malignant effusions. *Eur J Cardiothoracic Surg*. 200;18(2):143–146.

48. Ferguson AD, Prescott RJ, Selkon JB, Watson D, Swinburn CR. Empyema subcommittee of the Research Committee of the British Thoracic Society. The clinical course and management of thoracic empyema. *Q J Med*. 1996;89:285–289.

7
Pneumothorax in the Critically Ill

Mansoor Sange and Chris J. Langrish

Abstract Pneumothorax is a relatively frequent occurrence in the intensive care unit (ICU). It may be procedure-related, due to severe underlying pulmonary disease and/or baro/volutrauma from mechanical ventilation. Some conditions, such as the acute respiratory distress syndrome (ARDS), predispose patients to develop pneumothorax and multiple air leaks may arise in individual patients during the course of their admission. Pneumothorax can lead to significant morbidity, particularly when it is under tension. Diagnosis is challenging in the ICU environment, and relies on a combination of clinical skills and a number of different imaging modalities. Management involves drainage, implementation of a ventilatory strategy to minimize air leak and treatment of the underlying pulmonary disorder. Occasionally, surgical intervention—thoracoscopy, stapling of surface blebs, pleurodesis—may be required. Recurrence rates following such interventions are reported to be low.

Introduction

A pneumothorax is defined as a collection of air in the space between the visceral and parietal layers of the lung pleura.[1] The incidence of pneumothorax in mechanically ventilated patients has declined over the last 2 decades from around 20% to 3%[2,3], probably due to the dissemination of lung-protective ventilation strategies, however its occurrence often leads to significant morbidity. This may be explained in part by the loss of essential lung function in a group of patients with limited cardiorespiratory reserve, and the potential for a simple pneumothorax to develop into a life-threatening tension pneumothorax in those receiving positive pressure ventilation.

Classification and Aetiology

Pneumothorax may be classified as primary or secondary, depending on the absence/presence of underlying lung disease. Risk factors for primary pneumothorax include smoking, tall stature and some familial genes.

In the intensive care environment the most common aetiological factors are:

- Baro/volutrauma from mechanical ventilation
- Iatrogenic complication of an invasive procedure
- Underlying lung disease
- Trauma (Figure 7.1)

Use of excessive airway pressure (barotrauma) and/or tidal volume (volutrauma) are important aetiological factors in the development of pneumothoraces in mechanically ventilated patients, particularly in those with severe underlying lung disease such as acute respiratory distress syndrome (ARDS). Other pulmonary diseases associated with an increased risk of pneumothorax include chronic obstructive pulmonary disease, bullous emphysema, *Pneumocystis* pneumonia (PCP), cystic fibrosis and tuberculosis.[4] In these patients multiple, complex and repeated air leaks are often seen. Weight <80 kg, acquired immunodeficiency syndrome (AIDS) and cardiogenic pulmonary oedema at the time of admission have been identified as additional risk factors in a prospective cohort study.[5]

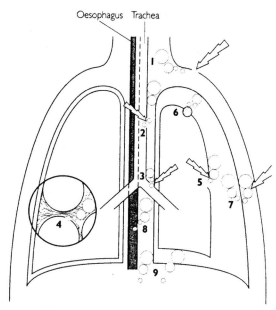

Oesophagus Trachea

⟁⟁⟁ True traumatic causes

FIGURE 7.1. Causes of air penetration into the pleura:
1. Soft tissue injury to the subclavian region
2. Trauma to the trachea
3. Trauma to the bronchus
4. Alveolar rupture
5. Rupture of the visceral pleura
6. Rupture of preformed bullae or blebs
7. Trauma to the external chest wall and parietal pleura
8. Rupture of the oesophagus
9. Entry of air from the abdomen

The procedures most commonly linked to inadvertent pneumothorax formation are thoracocentesis, central venous cannulation (subclavian > internal jugular approach), transbronchial biopsy and tracheostomy formation. The incidence of pneumothorax complicating thoracocentesis may be reduced by using ultrasound (US) to guide the procedure.[6]

Traumatic pneumothorax should be suspected and sought in cases of direct chest wall trauma, pulmonary contusion and diaphragmatic injury. In this situation the pneumothorax is said to be 'open' if it communicates with the exterior.

There are few data regarding prognostic factors and outcomes in critically ill patients, although pneumothorax associated with barotrauma, tension pneumothorax and concurrent sepsis is reported to carry a particularly bleak outlook.[3]

Patients with procedure-related pneumothorax tend to fare better, as demonstrated in a recent retrospective cohort study in which 59% of the pneumothoraces during a 3-year period were procedure-related.[3,7]

Pathophysiology

In many severe lung diseases, such as ARDS, there is direct tissue damage due to the host inflammatory response and/or toxins produced by the causative organism, e.g. Pneumocystis. Infarction can also occur as a result of local vascular compromise. Subpleural cysts or cavities form, which may eventually leak air. If this leak is significant, air will accumulate in the pleural space, usually towards the apex in a spontaneously breathing erect patient, due to the higher negative pressure in the pleural cavity (pleural pressure gradient increases from base to apex). This may remain a small localised collection or, depending on disease progression and airway pressure, increase in size resulting in loss of lung volume and impaired ventilation/perfusion matching. As the pressure in the affected hemithorax continues to rise the mediastinal structures, including major blood vessels, become compressed and shift towards the opposite side of the chest. Venous return is reduced and cardiac afterload increases. Cardiac output is usually severely reduced under these circumstances—known as a tension pneumothorax—and if the pleural air collection is not decompressed, it may promptly culminate in a cardiac arrest. Although ventilated patients with air leaks are at constant risk of this dangerous sequence of events, in reality, tension pneumothorax is uncommon. Most patients with air leaks develop localised collections which resolve, albeit slowly in patients with underlying pathology, after drainage.

Pneumothorax ex vacuo is a rare phenomenon, which occurs at the site of atelectatic obstructed lung or fixed trapped lung following drainage of an effusion. The rapid drainage of fluid combined with the inability of the lung parenchyma to re-expand leads to the generation of a negative intrapleural pressure which encourages the passage of nitrogen into the space from the local microcirculation leading to a collection.

Clinical Diagnosis and Imaging

Clinical Diagnosis

The classical findings on clinical examination in patients with a pneumothorax are:

- Decreased chest movement on the affected side
- Hyper resonance on percussion of the affected side
- Decreased or absent breath sounds on the affected side
- Hyperinflation of the affected side
- Tracheal deviation away from the affected side

Given the limitations of clinical examination in critically ill ventilated patients, clinicians must also be alert to other signs that may indicate the development of a pneumothorax:

- Worsening gas exchange or increased oxygen requirements
- A need for increased ventilatory support, raised peak airway pressures or abnormal respiratory pattern
- Cardiovascular changes such as tachycardia, hypotension or rising central venous pressure
- Evidence of decreased end-organ perfusion, e.g. metabolic acidosis (elevated lactate), oliguria

Misdiagnosis of pneumothorax is particularly common in critically ill patients who have an altered mental state, are receiving sedation, present out of hours or have atypical radiological findings.[8,9]

Imaging

Chest X-Ray (CXR)

This is the most frequently used modality in the diagnosis of pneumothorax, the gold-standard being the erect, posterior–anterior (P-A), expiratory film. Unfortunately, most critically ill patients will not be stable enough for transfer to the radiology department, and clinicians must therefore rely upon portable AP chest x-rays to assist in the diagnosis. In addition, it is often difficult to obtain an erect film due to haemodynamic instability or patient immobility, and a supine or semi-erect film may be the only practical option. Approximately 500 mL of pleural gas is needed for a definitive diagnosis of pneumothorax to be made.[10] CXR features include peripheral loss of bronchovascular lung markings (hyperlucency), and presence of a clear, white line demarcating the lung border medial to this. Hyperexpansion of the affected hemithorax may also be noted. The presence of a 'deep sulcus' sign at the diaphragm is useful in estimating the volume of the pneumothorax as a percentage of the hemithorax. Clinicians should be wary of conditions that can mimic pneumothorax, including large subpleural bullae, diaphragmatic herniae containing gas-filled bowel and excessive skin folds.[11]

Computed Tomography (CT) Scan

CT scan is a more sensitive and specific modality than CXR in the diagnosis of pneumothorax. It has a particularly important role in distinguishing bullous emphysema from pneumothorax, and in detecting multiple, unilateral pneumothoraces. It is not unusual in critically ill patients with unremarkable CXRs to detect a pneumothorax with CT imaging (Figure 7.2). CT scanning can also be extremely helpful in guiding the placement of chest drains. It is important to ensure that CT scanning is only attempted in those patients who are stable enough to undergo a transfer to the radiology department.

Ultrasound

Ultrasound may be useful in detecting occult pneumothoraces, and has been shown to reduce the need for CT scanning. Useful signs include the sliding lung, the 'A' sign and the lung point.[12,13] Although highly sensitive and specific in the right hands, it is very operator dependent. It plays a major role in real-time guidance of chest drain placement.

Endoscopy

Some clinicians recommend the routine use of thoracoscopy in the management of pneumothorax. It allows visualisation of bronchopleural fistulae, optimal drain placement and pleurodesis if required.

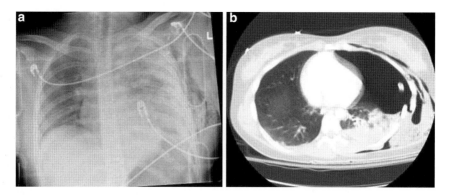

FIGURE 7.2. *Left*: Anterosuperior supine chest radiograph of a blunt trauma victim revealing left posterolateral rib fractures and parenchymal opacity due to pleural fluid and pulmonary contusion. There is no obvious pneumothorax. *Right*: CT scan reveals a large occult left-sided pneumothorax.

Management

There are three important aspects to managing a pneumothorax:

- Treatment of any underlying lung pathology
- Drainage of air from the pleural space
- Early detection and management of complications such as tension pneumothorax, persisting air leak, bronchopleural fistula (particularly prevalent in post-operative thoracic surgical patients) and infected pleural space (empyema)

Treatment of Any Underlying Lung Disease

If the pneumothorax is secondary to underlying lung disease, such as pneumonia, empyema, tuberculosis or ARDS, it is essential that appropriate medical and/or surgical management of that disease is instituted.

Drainage of Air from Pleural Space

A conservative approach may be used if the pneumothorax is small (<15%), and is not causing any significant symptoms. However, in mechanically ventilated patients there is a risk of tension pneumothorax, and a high level of awareness combined with frequent reassessments of the size of the pleural collection are mandatory. The pneumothorax will usually resorb spontaneously at a rate of 1.2–1.8% of the volume of the hemithorax per day, due to the gas tension gradient promoting diffusion of nitrogen from the pneumothorax into capillary blood. This gradient can be improved by administering increased levels of inspired oxygen.

Most patients with a significant air collection causing deterioration in their clinical state will require tube thoracostomy. A large bore (>20F) drain should be inserted in an aseptic manner using a blunt dissection technique and taking care to avoid using a trochar. This method minimises the risk of tube misplacement and possible damage to lung parenchyma, liver and spleen. The drain should be firmly sutured in place and attached to an underwater seal.

Smaller gauge Seldinger drains (12F), although less traumatic to insert, are generally unsuitable for patients undergoing positive pressure ventilation as their diameter may be insufficient to ensure adequate drainage of the pneumothorax. Since the incidence of misplacement is high with Seldinger drains, real-time US or CT imaging should be used to assist their insertion.

Suction should not be routinely applied to chest drains following elective lung surgery, since there is no evidence that it reduces the duration of air leak.[14] It may however be useful in individual cases. High-volume low-pressure systems are recommended (-10 to $-20\,cm\,H_2O$). Clinicians should be aware that application of suction in mechanically ventilated patients may result in increasing pneumothorax due to limitation of air flow by the suction system itself. In this situation, suction should be removed from the drain. Consideration should be given to the insertion of a second, larger drain if the problem remains unresolved.

In a minority of cases with multiple pneumothoraces due to severe underlying lung disease, e.g. ARDS, PCP, multiple chest drains may be required for several weeks. There is no evidence for routine tube changes; however, the drain site should be inspected daily for signs of local infection.

The chest drain is usually removed once the pneumothorax has resolved on CXR and there has been no air leakage for at least 24 h.

Early Detection and Management of Complications

The presence of surgical emphysema implies that an air-filled space is in communication with the tissues, and the chest drain should be checked for misplacement, kinking or blockage. The surgical emphysema itself is of cosmetic importance only, and will resolve over a few days once any problem with the drain has been rectified.

Infection of the pleural space (empyema) is more common in trauma cases. Rib resection may be required in addition to antibiotics and standard tube thoracostomy to achieve adequate drainage of the infected space.

In cases with persisting air leak, it is vital to ensure that any underlying lung disease is adequately treated. A number of ventilatory strategies aimed at minimising the size of the air leak may be tried including reducing tidal volume, respiratory frequency, positive end-expiratory pressure (PEEP) and inspiratory time. Other strategies include high frequency oscillatory ventilation (HFOV) or selective intubation of the unaffected lung and differential lung ventilation. In patients with continuing air leak despite these manoeuvres, video-assisted thoracic surgery (VATS) or open thoracotomy should be considered. Small surface blebs (<2 cm) can often be obliterated with laser or argon coagulation; however, larger blebs (>2 cm) will usually need surgical excision or stapling. This can be followed by pleurodesis using sclerosing agents or mechanical abrasion. Recurrence rates for pneumothorax following VATS are low.

Tension Pneumothorax

Tension pneumothorax is a relatively uncommon medical emergency; however, if it is unrecognised or left untreated can result in death. In patients receiving positive pressure ventilation the delivery of supra-physiological airway pressures can lead to a rapid dramatic decompensation.

Recent literature suggests that clinical presentation is remarkably consistent in ventilated patients, featuring a rapid and progressive deterioration in arterial and venous oxygenation combined with hypotension and a fall in cardiac output. High ventilatory pressures, lateralising signs such as decreased air entry and hyper-inflation are present in only about a third of cases. Other clinical signs, such as venous distension and surgical emphysema, are unreliable.

Delaying intervention in ventilated patients, in order to obtain a CXR, is associated with increased mortality and has led to the belief that radiography has no place in the diagnosis of tension pneumothorax. Whilst as a general rule this is true, each individual case should be considered on its own merits. It should be remembered that there are risks associated with both needle decompression and chest drain insertion (haemorrhage, tamponade, infection). Whilst radiography should never delay drainage in a deteriorating case with clinical suspicion of a tension pneumothorax, it may be useful in less acute situations.[15]

In ventilated patients, needle/cannnula decompression has a role in the emergency situation, but has a high failure rate due to obstruction/kinking, misplacement and an inability to drain large collections adequately. The traditional approach for needle/cannula decompression is though the 2nd/3rd intercostal space in the mid-clavicular line. However, this may fail if the pleural cavity is located deep below well-developed pectoral muscles.

Some recent guidelines have advocated the use of the 5th intercostal space in the mid-axillary line, a site containing less fat and avoiding muscle. The use of a syringe filled with normal saline may facilitate detection of the pleural space.

Chest drain insertion is the definitive treatment for a tension pneumothorax. It ensures adequate drainage of the pleural space and should result in re-expansion of the lung. Complications are now rare, since the implementation of blunt dissection with a 360° finger sweep, making use of a trochar unnecessary. Thoracostomy using blunt dissection without tube insertion is an alternative in the pre-hospital environment.

References

1. Henry M, Arnold T, Harvey J. BTS guidelines for the management of spontaneous pneumothorax. *Thorax.* 2003;58 Suppl 2:ii39–52.

2. Sassoon CS et al. Iatrogenic pneumothorax: etiology and morbidity. Results of a Department of Veterans Affairs cooperative study. *Respiration.* 2002;59(4): 215–220.

3. Chen KY, Jerng JS, Liao WY, Ding LW, Kuo LC, Wang JY, et al. Pneumothorax in the ICU: patient outcomes and prognostic factors. *Chest.* 2002;122(2):678–683.

4. Wait MA and Estrera A. Changing clinical spectrum of spontaneous pneumothorax. *Am J Surg.* 1992; 164(5):528–531.

5. de Lassence A, Timsit JF, Tafflet M, Azoulay E, Jamali S, Vincent F, et al. Pneumothorax in the intensive care unit: incidence, risk factors, and outcome. *Anesthesiology.* 2006;104(1):5–13.

6. Raptopoulos V, Davis LM, Lee G, Umali C, Lew R, Irwin RS. Factors affecting the development of pneumothorax associated with thoracentesis. *Am J Roentgenol.* 1991;156(5):917–920.

7. Despars JA, Sassoon CS, Light RW. Significance of iatrogenic pneumothoraces. *Chest.* 1994;105(4):1147–1150.

8. Kollef MH. Risk factors for the misdiagnosis of pneumothorax in the intensive care unit. *Crit Care Med.* 1991;19(7):906–910.

9. Kollef MH. The effect of an increased index of suspicion on the diagnosis of pneumothorax in the critically ill. *Mil Med.* 1992;157(11):591–593.

10. Carr JJ, Reed JC, Choplin RH, Pope TL Jr, Case LD. Plain and computed radiography for detecting experimentally induced pneumothorax in cadavers: implications for detection in patients. *Radiology.* 1992;183(1):193–199.

11. Rankine JJ, Thomas AN, Fluechter D. Diagnosis of pneumothorax in critically ill adults. *Postgrad Med J.* 2000;76(897):399–404.

12. Lichtenstein DA, Menu Y. A bedside ultrasound sign ruling out pneumothorax in the critically ill. Lung sliding. *Chest.* 1995;108(5):1345–1348.

13. Lichtenstein DA, Mezière G, Lascols N, Biderman P, Courret JP, Gepner A, et al. Ultrasound diagnosis of occult pneumothorax. *Crit Care Med.* 2005;33(6): 1231–1238.

14. Alphonso N, Tan C, Utley M, Cameron R, Dussek J, Lang-Lazdunski L, Treasure T. A prospective randomized controlled trial of suction versus non-suction to the under-water seal drains following lung resection. *Eur J Cardiothorac Surg.* 2005;27(3): 391–394.

15. Leigh-Smith S, Harris T. Tension time for a re-think. *Emerg Med J.* 2005;22:8–16.

8
Diagnosis and Management of the Obstructed Airway

Adrian Pearce and Gerard Gould

Abstract The obstructed airway presents a potentially life-threatening and terrifying (for both clinician and patient!) clinical situation. At all times a thorough assessment is required and highly skilled and experienced staff should be involved from an early stage. It is imperative that management is underpinned by a sound understanding of the possible underlying pathologies and the pitfalls associated with clinical intervention.

Introduction

The obstructed airway is the clinical situation in which a patient develops signs or symptoms due to narrowing or distortion of the airway. Narrowing of the airway increases the resistance to airflow and respiratory effort increases to maintain alveolar ventilation and gaseous homeostasis. Two broad clinical patterns, acute and chronic, can be recognised.

In acute airway obstruction, narrowing occurs in minutes, hours or a few days, and the untrained respiratory muscles tire easily. Alveolar ventilation cannot be sustained and the increasing levels of hypoxaemia and hypercapnia give rise to florid signs and symptoms of respiratory distress necessitating urgent intervention.

In chronic obstruction, narrowing or distortion develops over weeks or months and allows respiratory muscle training such that alveolar ventilation may be maintained even when the airway diameter is narrowed to less than 3 mm. Intervention is not immediately needed.

Acute Obstruction

Causes

The disease processes which distort the airway within minutes or hours are generally 'fluidic' in nature and involve oedema, blood, pus or a foreign body. The commonest site is 'upper airway', a rather ill-defined term which includes the glottis, supraglottis, tongue base and pharynx. Common causes of acute upper airway obstruction are

- Infections such as epiglottitis, retropharyngeal abscess or diphtheria
- Airway oedema due to anaphylaxis, angiotensin-converting enzyme inhibitors, angio-oedema or thermal injury
- Bleeding into a cyst (Figure 8.1) or postoperative haematoma in the head or neck
- Foreign body
- Airway trauma

Symptoms and Signs

With sudden complete airway obstruction the clinical presentation is as outlined below:

- Patient is unable to breath, speak or cough
- Patient may hold throat between thumb and index finger (universal choking sign)

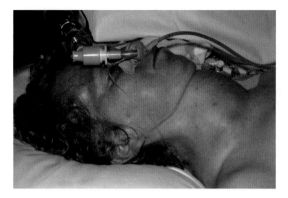

FIGURE 8.1. Bleeding into a thyroid cyst causing acute airway obstruction.

- Patient is anxious and agitated
- Patient may have progressed to loss of consciousness, bradycardia and hypoxia with a silent chest
- Death is inevitable if obstruction is not immediately relieved

In the setting of partial airway obstruction, symptoms and signs are due to increased work of breathing, ineffective alveolar ventilation and the secondary effects of hypoxia and hypercapnia.

- Hypoxaemia, tachypnoea, nasal flaring, use of accessory muscles, adoption of sitting position, tachycardia, sweating, anxiety, restlessness, depressed level of consciousness—due to the increased work of breathing or failure of gaseous homeostasis
- See-saw pattern of respiratory movements with intercostal and substernal recession
- Stridor (noisy breathing) due to narrowing of the airway lumen causing a change from laminar to turbulent airflow and hence noisy breathing. The airway diameter is said to be less than 50% if stridor is present and 4.5 mm or less if present at rest. If the lesion is above the vocal cords (extrathoracic), then the stridor will be inspiratory in nature. If the pathology is below the vocal cords (intrathoracic), then stridor will occur in the expiratory phase
- Difficulty in swallowing—indicates pharyngeal involvement
- Hoarse voice—laryngeal involvement
- Dribbling and retention of secretions

Diagnosis and Investigations

The diagnosis of acute airway obstruction is easy to make when the patient presents with noisy, difficult breathing. The aetiology may not be immediately obvious but is suggested by the history. Sudden onset suggests foreign body inhalation, which may be self-reported or witnessed and must always be considered in children. Prodromal sore throat and pyrexia suggests an infective cause and perusal of the medications will identify those on ACE inhibitors. Examination will reveal obvious masses, infections or trauma in the head or neck. Once the history and examination have been performed the following investigations may be considered to support the diagnosis and attempt to identify the site and extent of any pathology.

Investigations

- Chest x-ray (CXR) to estimate airway diameter, any obvious extrinsic compression, tracheal deviation, radio-opaque foreign body, obstructive emphysema and to exclude pneumothorax
- Radiographs of the soft tissues of the neck can be useful to detect radio-opaque foreign bodies, retropharyngeal masses and epiglottitis
- Computed tomography (CT)/magnetic resonance imaging (MRI) can be used in a stable patient. The integrity of the thyroid, cricoid and arytenoid cartilages as well as the status of the airway lumen can be assessed
- The supraglottis and glottis can be viewed and assessed by indirect mirror laryngoscopy or flexible fibre-optic nasendoscopy. It is very helpful to know if the vocal cords can be visualised and to assess if a tracheal tube will pass through the glottis

Three serious management pitfalls must be emphasised. Firstly, stridor is not always present and life-threatening obstruction may be 'silent'. Secondly, monitoring of oxygen saturations is not a useful method of identifying the seriousness of the situation. Figure 8.2 shows the relationship in a normal patient (with normal lungs) between the alveolar minute ventilation and arterial oxygen tension. It can be seen that while breathing air there will be a noticeable decline in oxygen saturation as alveolar minute ventilation decreases. Breathing high-inspired oxygen concentrations

FIGURE 8.2. Relationship between alveolar minute ventilation and alveolar PO_2.

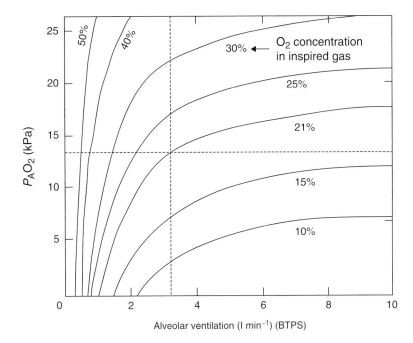

maintains an adequate arterial PO_2 even when alveolar minute ventilation is at very low levels. The seriousness of the situation must be assessed by the perceived work of breathing or arterial blood gas monitoring to measure pH and $PaCO_2$. Thirdly, a definite decision needs to be made as to whether a patient is well enough to undergo a diagnostic procedure such as x-ray or direct inspection of the pharynx. Sudden deterioration may ensue in an environment which is unsuitable for urgent airway intervention and the patient should be accompanied by a clinician competent at emergency airway intervention.

Management

Obstruction due to glottic impaction of a food-bolus should be treated by the Heimlich manoeuvre. On arrival at hospital, if airway obstruction is complete, attempts must be made to oxygenate and ventilate the patient and support the cardiovascular system. A rapid attempt at intubation is worthwhile, but may prove impossible and should not delay emergency cricothyrotomy or tracheostomy.

With partial airway obstruction it is important to involve experienced senior ENT (or maxillo-facial and thoracic) surgeons and anaesthetists. Treatment depends to a certain extent on the aetiology.

- Administer 100% oxygen by facemask
- Allow the patient to adopt the most comfortable position, usually sitting up
- Establish IV access and administer fluid resuscitation as appropriate. These patients will often be hypovolaemic, particularly if the disease process has affected oral intake or if the patient is pyrexial
- Minimum monitoring should include SaO_2, ECG and non-invasive blood pressure (NIBP)
- Nebulised epinephrine (adrenaline) in 100% oxygen, usually given in 1 mg aliquots up to a maximum of 5 mg. This can be very useful when the aetiology is one of airway oedema
- Parenteral epinephrine (adrenaline) 1:10,000 may be required where airway obstruction is part of a general anaphylactoid reaction
- Consider a trial of Heliox (79% helium and 21% oxygen) for symptomatic relief where large airway narrowing is associated with turbulent flow. The low density of helium is favourable in turbulent flow
- Steroid administration, hydrocortisone 200 mg IV, is also useful in minimising airway oedema, but will not be effective for a number of hours
- Antibiotic administration for infection, usually a broad-spectrum penicillin plus metronidazole if anaerobic infection (such as a dental abscess) is suspected

- Consider arterial cannulation in the more serious or rapidly developing situation. A rising $PaCO_2$ and falling pH are indicators that airway support will be needed
- High dependency unit (HDU) or intensive care unit (ICU) is the appropriate environment for continuing treatment and supervised transfer should be organised

Failure of conservative management is indicated by increasing respiratory effort or fatigue, decrease in level of consciousness or worsening blood gases. Airway intervention is required and often proves to be difficult.

- Pre-existing airway obstruction is likely to be worsened by lying the patient flat, by instrumentation of the larynx or by the use of general anaesthesia
- Identifying the laryngeal inlet may be difficult because of anatomical distortion, particularly with supraglottic lesions or airway oedema
- Severe stenosis may limit intubation, particularly at glottic or subglottic level

Airway Intervention Strategies

It is important to work out a plan for airway management under the guidance of senior anaesthetists and surgeons. There are no proven ideal techniques but an assessment of the safest, most familiar approach should be made. There needs to be a primary plan (plan A) with a default back-up plan (plan B) that can be implemented by the personnel available. Whichever technique is used, a full range of equipment should be prepared including different laryngoscopes, various sized endotracheal tubes (ETTs), cricothyrotomy equipment and facilities for surgical tracheostomy.

There are four main approaches that can be adopted and each has its benefits and potential pitfalls:

1. Tracheostomy under local anaesthesia
2. Awake fibreoptic intubation
3. General anaesthesia and intubation or tracheostomy
4. Emergency cricothyrotomy

Tracheostomy Under Local Anaesthesia

- Where mask ventilation is predicted to be difficult and awake fibreoptic intubation is contraindicated or not possible

- Can be very difficult in the agitated, hypoxic patient who cannot lie flat
- May be technically difficult due to distorted anatomy
- Avoid sedative agents as this can precipitate complete obstruction

Awake Fibreoptic Intubation

- Technically challenging in this group of patients
- It should be performed by an anaesthetist experienced in fibreoptic techniques and in the management of patients with airway obstruction
- Most useful in patients whose pathology is above normal vocal cords
- Give an antisialogogue and perform the procedure in the sitting position
- Sedation is contraindicated and applying topical anaesthesia to the vocal cords can precipitate laryngeal spasm. As a result the procedure should be carried out in the operating theatre with a tracheostomy set and senior surgeon scrubbed and ready
- If the lesion is at the glottic or subglottic level, then there may be difficulty railroading an ETT over the fibrescope or complete obstruction may occur (Figure 8.3a–c)

General Anaesthesia and Intubation or Tracheostomy

Generally, induction of anaesthesia should be undertaken in the operating theatre with a surgeon ready to perform urgent tracheostomy if intubation fails. Both inhalational and intravenous induction of anaesthesia has been promoted with no clear consensus. The major arguments for and against each technique are:

- Inhalational induction of anaesthesia (Figure 8.4) with 8% sevoflurane in 100% oxygen allows retention of spontaneous ventilation and is reversible in the early stages, so that if problems occur it can be stopped and an awake tracheostomy performed
- It is difficult to achieve deep anaesthesia with inhalational induction in cases of airway obstruction and laryngeal spasm may be provoked under light plains of general anaesthesia
- When using sevoflurane, hypoventilation and apnoea are not uncommon
- Intravenous induction provides rapid loss of consciousness, low oxygen consumption by the

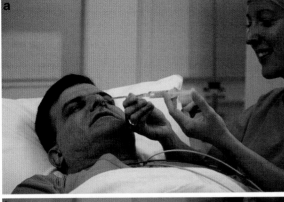

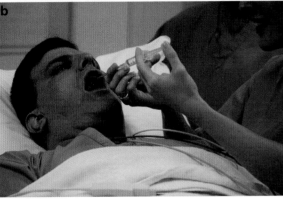

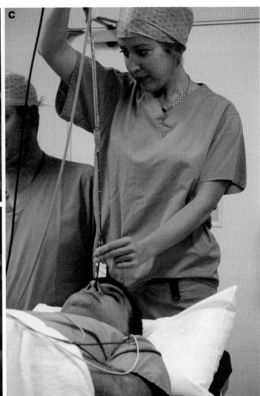

FIGURE 8.3. Awake fibre-optic intubation. (**a**) Topical anaesthesia nares. (**b**) Topical anaesthesia oro pharynx. (**c**) Awake fibre-optic intubation.

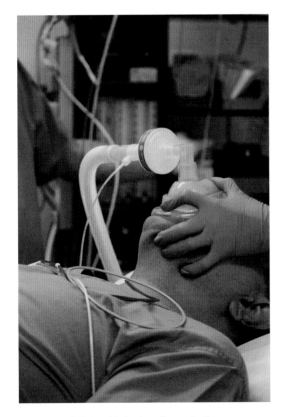

FIGURE 8.4. Inhalational induction of anaesthesia.

body, good conditions for an attempt at direct laryngoscopy or for urgent tracheostomy

- Intravenous induction abolishes spontaneous respiration and muscle tone and may precipitate a 'can't ventilate, can't intubate' (CVCI) scenario

The laryngeal mask (LMA) has proved useful in maintaining the airway in some anaesthetised or unconscious patients with upper airway obstruction and may maintain a satisfactory airway while tracheostomy is undertaken. Another technique gaining popularity is the placement of a trans-tracheal ventilation catheter through the cricothyroid membrane (CTM) or trachea in the awake patient prior to induction of anaesthesia (Figure 8.5a and b). This catheter may be used for oxygenation of the patient during intubation or tracheostomy. Such a catheter can be considered only if the level of obstruction is known to be above the catheter insertion point. The correct position of the catheter should be confirmed by free aspiration of air and capnography prior to use. It needs to be secured in place and, if ventilation with high-pressure oxygen is required, particular attention is needed to avoid barotrauma.

a b

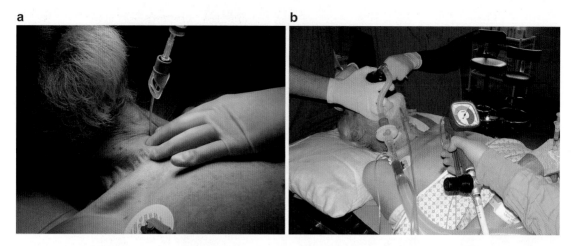

FIGURE 8.5. (a) Transtracheal catheter placed under local anaesthesia. (b) Attachment of high-pressure oxygen to cannula.

Emergency Cricothyrotomy

Emergency cricothyrotomy may be needed at any time to provide oxygenation when the normal airway fails. The cricothyroid membrane has a number of desirable features, but the upper trachea is also a suitable location.

The cricothyroid membrane (CTM) has the following characteristics:

- Present in most patients and rarely calcifies
- Easy to locate and relatively superficial
- Relatively avascular
- One centimetre below the vocal cords
- Approximately 8 mm below the skin in the midline
- Is 9–10 mm high and 22–30 mm wide
- The complete cricoid ring provides support during catheter insertion
- The posterior lamina of the cricoid cartilage decreases the chance of damage to the posterior tracheal wall

There are three types of cricothyrotomy—small needle or cannula (Figure 8.6), large (>4 mm diameter) purpose-built cannula (Figure 8.7) and a surgical tube (6 mm diameter). The small cannula is inserted through the CTM and angled caudad into the trachea (Figure 8.8 a–d). Its narrow diameter and high resistance to airflow necessitate high-pressure oxygen at 2–4 bar to provide effective ventilation. Exhalation occurs through the upper airway

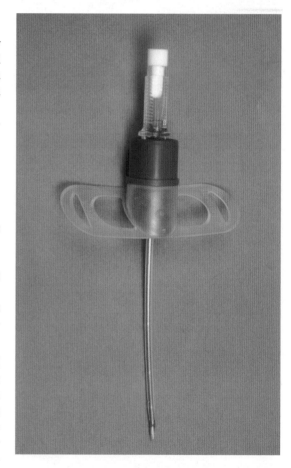

FIGURE 8.6. Small 13 Ga cricothyrotomy cannula ~2 mm internal diameter.

FIGURE 8.7. Large cricothyrotomy cannula >4 mm internal diameter.

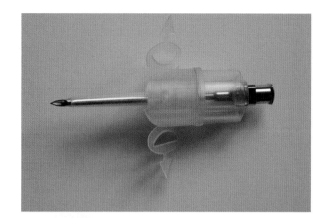

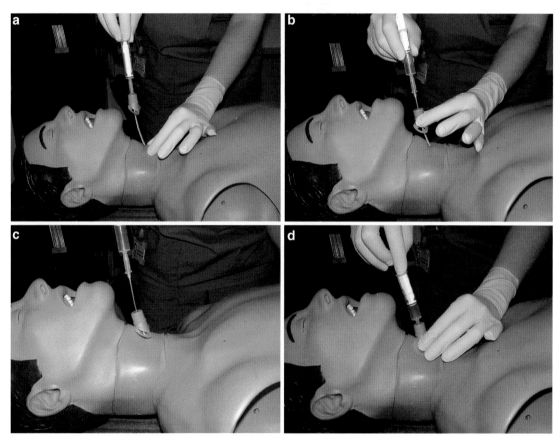

FIGURE 8.8. (**a–d**). Steps in placement of a small cannula cricothyrotomy.

and barotrauma is possible. The large purpose-built cannula (>4 mm) allows use of the standard breathing system and exhalation occurs through the cannula. Surgical cricothyrotomy enables direct placement of a 6 mm tube into the trachea.

Chronic Obstruction

Where the disease process develops relatively slowly over weeks or months, the respiratory muscle adaptation allows maintenance of normal

FIGURE 8.9. Large goitre.

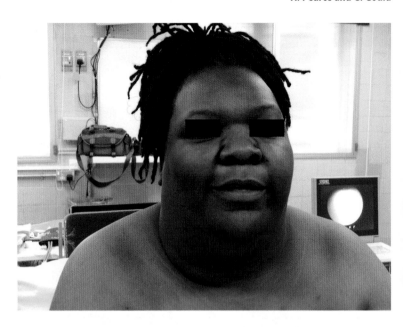

alveolar ventilation until the airway is narrowed to only a few millimetres in diameter. Generally the disease process is a benign or malignant tumour, chronic inflammation such as Wegener's granulomatosis, fibrosis due to surgery or radiotherapy or stenosis due to prolonged intubation or tracheostomy.

At rest, patients may have few symptoms but are generally short of breath on exertion. They may have a position in which breathing is optimum and they may exhibit symptoms such as voice change or dysphagia related to the disease process causing obstruction. Signs of increased respiratory work may not be evident and the increased respiratory muscle bulk cannot be seen. There may be an obvious mass such as a goitre (Figure 8.9). There are often subtle changes in timbre of voice, strength of cough or a 'rasping' noise on respiration.

The most important aspect of management is MRI or CT imaging from the base of skull to carina and flexible nasendoscopy to delineate the extent and degree of airway narrowing. Flow-volume loops as part of pulmonary function tests can help identify the site of airway obstruction. The pathology indicates whether the narrowing is likely to be fixed or amenable to passage of a reasonable sized tracheal tube. Surgical intervention may be required for biopsy or debulking of a tumour, dilatation of a stenotic section or excision of a mass impinging on the airway.

Central Airway Obstruction

Central airway obstruction refers to the scenario where the obstruction, usually an intrinsic or extrinsic tumour, affects the lower trachea and carina. This region is beyond the reach of standard tracheostomy tubes or emergency oxygenation by cricothyrotomy. Unrecognised anterior mediastinal masses are one cause of catastrophic failure of ventilation after induction of anaesthesia. Where possible, imaging of the airway allows planning of surgical and anaesthetic intervention. Standard tracheal tubes may not pass the obstruction and a rigid bronchoscope may be required. Occasionally, intubation of one bronchus and one lung ventilation is all that may be possible and this is maintained for several days during chemoradiotherapy. At other times tracheobronchial stents are effective. Surgical resection at the level of the lower trachea and carina is highly specialised work.

Further Reading

1. Chandradeva K, Palin C, Ghosh SM, Pinches SC (2005) Percutaneous transtracheal jet ventilation as a guide to tracheal intubation in severe upper airway obstruction from supraglottic oedema. British Journal of Anaesthesia 94:683–686.
2. Conacher I (2003) Anaesthesia and tracheobronchial stenting for central airway obstruction in adults. British Journal of Anaesthesia 90:367–374.

3. Gerig HJ, Schnider T, Heidegger T (2005) Prophylactic percutaneous transtracheal catheterisation in the management of patients with anticipated difficult airways: a case series. Anaesthesia 60:801–805.
4. Maloney E, Meakin GH (2007) Acute Stridor in children. Continuing Education in Anaesthesia, Critical Care & Pain 7:183–186.
5. Mason RA, Fielder CP (1999) The obstructed airway in head and neck surgery. Anaesthesia 54:625–628.
6. Ovassapian A, Tuncbilek M, Weitzel EK, Joshi CW (2005) Airway management in adult patients with deep neck infections: a case series and review of the literature. Anesthesia Analgesia 100:585–589.
7. Patel B, Frerk C (2008) Large-bore cricothyrotomy devices. Continuing Education in Anaesthesia, Critical Care & Pain 8:157–160.
8. Popat M, Dudnikov S (2001) Management of the obstructed upper airway. Current Anaesthesia and Critical Care 12:225–230.
9. Rees L, Mason RA (2002) Advanced upper airway obstruction in ENT surgery. Continuing Education in Anaesthesia, Critical Care & Pain 2:134–138.

9
Postoperative Management of Patients Undergoing Lung Resection, Oesophagectomy or Thymectomy

Michael Gillies and Paul Hayden

Abstract Patients undergoing thoracic and oesophageal surgery frequently have pre-existing cardiorespiratory and other general medical problems. This, combined with the nature of the surgery, makes their perioperative care extremely challenging. In this chapter the nature and management of postoperative complications are discussed. The importance of good analgesia and careful fluid balance are emphasised. Paravertebral block (PVB) is recommended for postoperative analgesia, since it has a better side-effect profile than thoracic epidural, and reduces pulmonary complications. Specific issues relating to oesophagectomy and thymectomy are also considered.

Introduction

This chapter outlines the basic principles of caring for the thoracic surgical patient during the postoperative period in the overnight intensive recovery unit (OIRU), high dependency unit (HDU) or intensive care unit (ICU) setting. The management of patients following oesophagectomy or thymectomy is given specific consideration, although many of the general postoperative issues in thoracic surgery will also apply in these cases.

Thoracic Surgery

General Considerations

The thoracic surgical patient frequently has pre-existing cardiorespiratory and other general medical problems. Pain and poor respiratory function following surgery may compound these problems, and result in severely impaired ventilation, decreased functional residual capacity (FRC) and sputum retention. These patients are therefore at high risk of perioperative complications, especially respiratory failure. Careful patient selection and meticulous care are essential if complications are to be minimised.[1]

In uncomplicated thoracic surgical cases, the patient is usually extubated in the operating theatre at the end of the procedure. Good analgesia is vital as it allows deep breathing, coughing and may attenuate the decrease in FRC. The patient is then transferred to the recovery area and nursed upright with supplemental oxygen. Intra-arterial blood pressure monitoring is often continued into the postoperative period, as this facilitates close observation of blood pressure and serial measurement of arterial blood gases. Occasionally, a period of ventilation is required postoperatively, especially in the frail, elderly or high-risk patient. This allows time for rewarming, optimisation of fluid status and correction of any acid–base or metabolic abnormality. If a period of postoperative ventilation is required it should be kept to a minimum, and high peak airway pressures avoided in order to prevent barotrauma to the bronchial stump and other anastamoses.

Routine investigations in the postoperative period include arterial blood gases, urea and electrolytes, full blood count and coagulation studies. A chest x-ray is essential and special attention should be paid to:

- Position of drains, tubes and intravascular catheters
- Lung expansion
- Presence of pneumothorax, haemothorax or other pleural collections
- Contour and position of mediastinal structures

Figure 9.1 is an example of a postoperative chest x-ray in a patient who has undergone a pneumonectomy.

Chest Drainage

Chest drains enable air or fluid (including blood) to escape from the pleural space, allow the lung to re-expand and prevent mediastinal shift. They are often, although not always, present in patients who have undergone thoracotomy.

A chest drainage system consists of an intercostal catheter and a collection system. Suction, if indicated, may also be added. A size 26 French gauge (Fr) catheter is commonly used in the postoperative setting, but sizes 24–36 Fr are available for use in adults, with the larger sizes usually reserved for drainage of blood or pus. The catheter is attached to the collection system by a length of PVC tubing, which ends 2 cm below the fluid level in the container. This underwater seal forms a one-way valve, allowing air and fluid to drain out of the pleural cavity while preventing the entry of air. Providing the container is kept below the patient, the seal cannot be broken during normal respiration and minimal resistance is offered to

the escape of air. Incremental markings on the side of the container allow estimation of blood or fluid loss (Figure 9.2).

Low-pressure suction may be applied to the collection system (usually at a level of 5 cmH$_2$O). Recent evidence suggests that routine application of suction is not necessary in patients following thoracotomy or video-assisted thoracoscopic surgery (VATS); however, it may assist with re-expansion of the lung and evacuation of air, fluid or blood.[2] Addition of positive end-expiratory pressure (PEEP) in mechanically ventilated patients may also promote lung re-expansion.

Classically, two drains are inserted following lung resection: an apical drain to remove air and a basal drain for the removal of fluid. Another approach is to insert two apical drains (anterior and posterior) with side holes to drain blood or fluid basally. If significant bleeding is unlikely no drains may be placed. Drains are removed when the lung has re-expanded radiologically, drainage of fluid and bubbling has ceased and there is minimal respiratory 'swing' of the fluid level. Following pneumonectomy, the drain is removed on the first postoperative day, allowing the pneumonectomy space to fill with exudate. The drain is removed with the patient performing a valsalva manoeuvre at full inspiration to minimise any influx of air. The wound is sutured, or if mattress sutures are already in place they are pulled tight, and an occlusive dressing is placed over the wound. A further chest radiograph is undertaken to exclude pneumothorax.

Persistent air leak may be problematic in the postoperative period, and if the volume is large surgical re-exploration may be required. Continu-

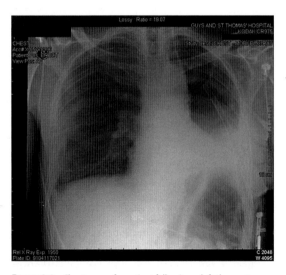

FIGURE 9.1. Chest x-ray of a patient following a left thoracotomy.

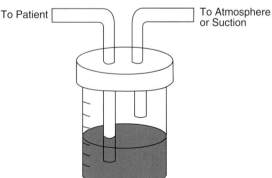

FIGURE 9.2. Schematic representation of a chest drainage system.

ing air leak is especially troublesome if the patient is mechanically ventilated, as a large proportion of the tidal volume may be lost through the chest drain and result in failure of ventilation and a rising arterial pCO_2. High-frequency oscillation can be used to overcome this problem if the air leak is large.

Postoperative Analgesia

Provision of good analgesia following thoracotomy is vital, enabling the patient to be extubated in the operating theatre, breathe deeply and cough. It minimises the reduction in FRC that occurs in the postoperative period, and reduces the incidence of pulmonary complications such as atelectasis and infection. While regional analgesia provides the cornerstone of postoperative analgesia in these cases, a 'multimodal' approach with frequent input from the acute pain service produces the best results (Table 9.1).

Paravertebral Block

Paravertebral block (PVB) is a mode of regional analgesia that can be delivered continuously via a paravertebral catheter or given as a 'single shot' injection, and has been shown to reduce pulmonary complications following thoracic surgery.[3] Although PVB and thoracic epidural analgesia (TEA) provide comparable pain relief, PVB has a better side-effect profile, and is the technique of choice in our institution in combination with patient-controlled analgesia (PCA).

TABLE 9.1. Analgesia following thoractomy

Regional techniques
- *Paravertebral block*: e.g. bupivacaine 0.25% 2–8 mL/h or 0.5% Lignocaine 10–12 mL/h
- *Epidural analgesia*: e.g. 0.1% bupivacaine with fentanyl 2 mcg/mL at 5–15 mL/h
- *Intrapleural analgesia*: e.g. bupivacaine 0.25% 2–8 mL/h
- *Intercostal nerve blocks*: e.g. 5 mL 0.5% bupivacaine with adrenaline 1 in 200,000 per segment

Opioid analgesia
- *Patient-controlled analgesia*: e.g. morphine 1 mg bolus, 5 min lockout

Non-steroidal anti-inflammatory drugs: e.g. diclofenac 50 mg 8 hourly

Adjunctive analgesics
- Ketamine i.v. infusion 5–20 mcg/kg/h
- Tramadol 50 mg 6 hourly
- Clonidine 2 mcg/kg

Thoracic Epidural

TEA is still widely used to minimise pain following thoracotomy, with a mixture of opioid and local anaesthetic usually being infused into the epidural space.

It has the advantage of offering a number of non-analgesic benefits, including reduced incidence of tachyarrhythmia, improved left ventricular function and reduced atelectasis and postoperative respiratory failure.

Other Regional Techniques

A number of other regional techniques may be used in post-thoracotomy patients. An intrapleural catheter, inserted at the time of surgery and positioned between the visceral and parietal pleura, can be used to deliver local anaesthetic postoperatively. However, the analgesic effect is often unpredictable with this technique, since local anaesthetic may be lost through drains or absorbed systemically. Intercostal nerve blocks provide limited short-term pain relief to areas supplied by the anterior rami of the intercostal nerves and can be delivered using a catheter-based or 'single shot' technique.

Systemic Analgesia

Although not the technique of choice for post-thoracotomy pain relief, patient-controlled analgesia with morphine or fentanyl is still used where regional techniques are refused or contraindicated. When administered and monitored correctly it can offer adequate pain relief; however, the incidences of respiratory depression, nausea and sedation are significant. Opioid analgesia can be supplemented with other drugs, notably non-steroidal anti-inflammatory drugs (NSAIDs), although these should be avoided in the elderly and those with a history of renal impairment. Ketamine and clonidine may also have a role in the treatment of breakthrough pain. Tramadol, with its lower incidence of respiratory depression, is a useful alternative to opioids.

Fluid Management

Surgical trauma, retraction, repeated collapse/re-expansion and overinflation can predispose patients to develop pulmonary oedema in the postoperative period. Fluid overload may also contribute to this, and it is prudent to avoid excessive volumes of crystalloid in these patients. Positive crystalloid balance should not exceed 20 mL/kg in the first postoperative day, and colloid or blood should be used to treat intravascular depletion where possible.

Postoperative Complications

Respiratory Failure

Patients undergoing thoracic surgery have a high incidence of coexisting respiratory disease, particularly a history of smoking, chronic obstructive pulmonary disease and occupational lung disease. Pain, obesity, supine positioning and pulmonary oedema may all contribute to postoperative respiratory failure. Good analgesia, upright posture, humidification of inspired gases, bronchodilator therapy and regular physiotherapy will help to minimise postoperative hypoxia. Sputum retention can be problematic in post-thoracotomy patients. If predicted postoperative FEV_1 is < 1 L, it is unlikely that the patient will be able to cough well enough to clear their own secretions. Phrenic nerve damage or partial chest wall resection may also contribute to ineffective coughing. Provision of good analgesia and physiotherapy are the mainstays of therapy. If sputum clearance remains problematic and respiratory failure ensues, a period of ventilation may be necessary. Tracheostomy may be helpful in a small number of patients requiring prolonged respiratory support and assistance with sputum clearance.

Acute lung injury following pneumonectomy has been described in a small percentage of patients undergoing lobectomy or pneumonectomy, and is also referred to as post-pneumonectomy or post-lung resection pulmonary oedema. Its aetiology is thought to be multifactorial. Surgical trauma and hyperinflation of the lung during one-lung ventilation may play a role, leading to neutrophil activation and formation of reactive oxygen species (ROS).[4] In common with other types of acute lung injury, high inflation pressures and tidal volumes should be avoided, and careful fluid management in the postoperative period is important. Both non-invasive ventilation (NIV) and intermittent continuous positive airway pressure (CPAP) have been used to improve gas exchange in this group of patients and may reduce the need for and duration of mechanical ventilation.

Blood Loss

Blood loss following thoracotomy varies according to the site and nature of the surgery. If drains are present blood loss can be measured objectively. Losses are often high in the first postoperative hour and rolling or turning the patient can result in a 'dump' of blood into the drain from the pleural cavity. Such blood loss is usually short-lived. Beyond this, ongoing losses of greater than 2 mL/kg/h are a cause for concern. Coagulopathy should be sought and treated and the surgical team informed. If drains are not present, a chest x-ray may reveal evidence of ongoing bleeding.

Dysrhythmias

Atrial fibrillation is common following thoracic surgical procedures. Any obvious precipitants such as hypoxia, hypokalaemia or hypomagnesaemia should be treated. If there is associated serious haemodynamic compromise DC cardioversion or administration of intravenous amiodarone may be required. Otherwise rate control can be achieved with digoxin or a beta blocker (unless contraindicated). Ventricular and other dysrhythmias are treated according to current life support guidelines.

Myocardial Ischaemia

Ischaemic heart disease is a common co-morbidity in this group of patients. It is important that anti-anginal and antihypertensive therapy is continued up to the day of surgery and recommended as soon as possible afterwards. There is some evidence that perioperative beta blockade, (provided that it is not contraindicated), may reduce the incidence of ischaemic events. Postoperative hypertension can be treated with an intravenous infusion of nitrates or beta blockers, e.g. GTN, labetolol.

Renal Failure

Pre-existing renal dysfunction, hypotension, hypovolaemia and the use of nephrotoxic drugs such as aminoglycosides and NSAIDS may all contribute to the development of postoperative renal failure. Optimising intravascular volume is particularly challenging in this group of patients, since fluid overload is poorly tolerated, and excessive volumes of crystalloid should certainly be avoided. The use of loop diuretics does not prevent the progression of renal dysfunction to frank failure, but is advocated by some to assist with fluid balance. There is no evidence to support the use of renal-dose dopamine.

Infection

The vast majority of patients are given 24 h of prophylactic perioperative antibiotics according to local policy. Further antibiotic therapy should be instituted if there is proven or suspected infection (e.g. purulent sputum, fever, rising inflammatory markers, new changes on chest x-ray). As always, antibiotic use should be guided by appropriate microbiological cultures.

Oesophagectomy

Despite advances in radiotherapy and chemotherapy, oesophagectomy still has a major role in managing patients with carcinoma of the oesophagus. In the past postoperative mortality was depressingly high, but recent data suggest that a 30-day mortality rate of 2–5% and 5-year survival approaching 30% can be achieved. This improvement is attributed to advances in postoperative intensive care management and centralisation of oesophageal surgery in 'high-volume' tertiary centres. Preoperative risk factors for mortality have been identified and include age, lung function, arterial blood gases, chronic respiratory disease and pre-existing liver disease. Patients may be risk stratified into three groups using the scoring system developed by Bartel[5] (Table 9.2).

The procedure itself is performed by a transthoracic or transhiatal approach. With the transthoracic approach, a right-sided thoracotomy is required for tumours in the upper two thirds of the oesophagus and a left-sided thoracotomy for those in the lower third. The transhiatal approach is predominantly for palliative resection of tumours below the carina, and carries a reduced incidence of respiratory compromise postoperatively but a higher incidence of anastamotic leakage.

Since cancer of the oesophagus is associated with poor nutrition, smoking and high alcohol intake, patients presenting for surgery often have

TABLE 9.2. Bartels risk stratification system for oesophageal surgery[4]

System	Normal	Compromised	Severely impaired
General status	4	8	12
Cardiovascular	3	6	9
Pulmonary	2	4	6
Hepatic	2	4	6

Score	Risk	30-day mortality (%)
11–15	Low	2
16–21	Moderate	5
22–33	High	25

poor cardiovascular, respiratory and nutritional status. These may be compounded by swallowing difficulties as a result of tumour bulk. Immunosuppression due to prior radiotherapy or chemotherapy may also predispose them to develop perioperative infection. In our institution anaerobic threshold, which has been shown to accurately predict postoperative mortality, is measured preoperatively and used to risk-stratify cases.

Respiratory failure occurs in approximately 25% of patients following oesophagectomy, and acute respiratory distress syndrome (ARDS) in 10–20%. Mortalities as high as 70% have been reported for post-oesophagectomy ARDS; however, it should be remembered that these data preceded publication of the ARDS Net study, following which changes in ventilator management have led to a general decrease in ARDS-related mortality.[6] The pathogenesis of lung injury following oesophagectomy is probably multifactorial. Collapse and re-expansion of the non-dependant lung during the procedure is associated with diffuse damage to the alveolar/epithelial interface, and is compounded by relative overventilation and barotrauma of the dependent lung. Subsequently, there is infiltration by inflammatory cells and increased vascular permeability resulting in ARDS. Bacterial translocation and endotoxin release from the gut may also be implicated in this process. Increased extravascular lung water due to volume loading perioperatively can compound the problem. A recent study identified low preoperative body mass index (BMI), history of smoking, haemodynamic instability intra-operatively, duration of surgery, need for re-operation and surgical experience as risk factors for the development of ARDS.

However, the most significant risk factor was anastamotic breakdown. Atelectasis, pleural effusions, pneumothoraces and pneumonia may all further complicate the postoperative course.

Many centres electively ventilate the patient overnight postoperatively using lung protective strategies to minimise pulmonary complications. Although immediate extubation is becoming more popular, a period of postoperative ventilation allows optimisation of analgesia, temperature and fluid balance. The patient should be extubated when fully alert and sitting upright to minimise risk of aspiration.

Careful fluid management is essential and vasopressor usage should be avoided if possible or kept to a minimum to protect the surgical anastamosis. Arrhythmias are common and electrolyte disturbances should be attended to quickly. Epidural analgesia is the cornerstone of pain relief. Early enteral nutrition, usually via a jejunostomy is also important, particularly to promote wound healing and maintain anastamotic integrity. Conversion to parenteral nutrition should not be delayed in cases of prolonged ileus or jejeunal tube displacement.

Thymectomy

Myaesthenia Gravis (MG) is an autoimmune disease characterised by weakness and fatigue of voluntary muscle. Patients often present initially with ptosis and visual disturbance. There is marked reduction of acetylcholine receptors at the neuromuscular junction and circulating anti-acetylcholine receptor antibodies are found in 85–90% of those with generalised disease. Therapy with anticholinesterase drugs provides temporary symptomatic relief, but many patients require immunosuppression with corticosteroids or immunosuppressant drugs. Plasma exchange or intravenous immunoglobulin provides short-term relief for those suffering from severe weakness or myaesthenic crisis.

Thymectomy is a widely accepted therapy for myaesthenic patients, particularly those with thymoma and early onset generalised MG. Although the efficacy of thymectomy is based on retrospective data, about 75% of patients obtain benefit from this procedure. Thymectomy can be undertaken from transcervical or suprasternal approaches. Usually, a limited median sternotomy is sufficient, although in severe hyperplasia a full sternotomy may be indicated.

TABLE 9.3. Scoring system used to predict the need for postoperative ventilation in patients with Myasthenia Gravis[7]

Patient factors	Points
Duration of disease >6 years	12
Coexisting respiratory disease	10
Pyridostigmine dose > 750 mg/day	8
Vital capacity <3 L	4

Score of ≥10 has a positive predictive value of 80%.

Mechanical ventilation is usually continued post-thymectomy in the OIRU or ICU. This provides additional time for the effects of muscle relaxants and anaesthetic agents to wear off. Opioids can be used in reduced doses to provide analgesia. Anticholinesterase therapy should be re-instituted at the preoperative level. Few patients require prolonged ventilation. Leventhal et al. (1980) devised a scoring system to predict the need for postoperative ventilatory support in patients undergoing trans-sternal thymectomy[7] (Table 9.3). Extubation is performed when the patient is awake, responsive and able to generate a pressure of $-20 \text{ cmH}_2\text{O}$.

References

1. Alphonso N, Tan C, Utley M, Cameron R, Dussek J, Lang-Lazdunski, L, et al. A prospective randomized controlled trial of suction versus non-suction to the under-water seal drains following lung resection. *Eur J Cardiothorac Surg.* 2005;27(3):391–394.
2. Avendano CE, Flume PA, Silvestri GA, King LB, Reed CE. Pulmonary complications after oesophagectomy. *Ann Thorac Surg.* 2002;73(3):922–926.
3. Benumof JL, Alfery DD. Anaesthesia for thoracic surgery. In: Miller RD, ed. *Anaesthesia.* 5th ed. New York: Churchill Livingston; 2000:1665–752.
4. Bartels H, Stein HJ, Siewert JR. Preoperative risk analysis and postoperative mortality of oesophagectomy for resectable oesophageal cancer. *Br J Surg.* 1998;85(6):840–844.
5. Davies RG, Myles PS, Graham JM. A comparison of the analgesic efficacy and side-effects of paravertebral vs epidural blockade for thoracotomy—a systematic review and meta-analysis of randomized trials. *Br J Anaesth.* 2006;96(4):418–426.
6. Grichnik KP. Acute lung injury and acute respiratory distress syndrome after pulmonary resection. *Semin Cardiothorac Vasc Anaesth.* 2004;8(4): 317–334.
7. Leventhal et al. Scoring system to predict need for postoperative ventilation in Myaesthenia Gravis. *Anaesthesiology.* 1980;53:26–30.

10
Indications for Ventilatory Support in Adults

David Goldhill

Abstract This chapter oulines the indications for intubation and ventilatory support in adults. A range of ventilatory options, both non-invasive and invasive, are described and their merits in specific clinical situations discussed.

Overview of Ventilatory Support in Adults

Mechanical ventilatory support is most commonly delivered through a tracheal tube or tracheostomy using a device that generates intermittent positive pressure.[1] Other options for support include non-invasive positive pressure ventilation (NIPPV), negative pressure ventilation (NPV) and a range of high-frequency ventilation techniques. There are many modes of positive pressure ventilation ranging from those which decrease the work of breathing and prevent airways collapse (e.g. continuous positive airway pressure [CPAP], bi-level positive airway pressure [BiPAP]), to those that provide more support and supplement spontaneous ventilation (e.g. pressure support [PS], synchronised intermittent mandatory ventilation [SIMV]) and those which fully support ventilation (e.g. continuous mandatory ventilation [CMV], inverse ratio ventilation [IRV]).

The physiological objectives of ventilation are to provide alveolar ventilation for the delivery of oxygen and removal of carbon dioxide, to expand the lung sufficiently to prevent or treat atelecta-sis, to maintain functional residual capacity (FRC), and to reduce the work of breathing such as in a patient with increased airways resistance or reduced compliance.[2,3] Mechanical ventilation is required when a patient's breathing is compromised because of neurological, muscular or anatomical causes, or when there is a failure of gas exchange because of problems with diffusion or ventilation perfusion mismatch. It may also be indicated to decrease systemic or myocardial oxygen consumption in patients with a high respiratory demand and compromised supply. Manipulation of $PaCO_2$ may be useful to control intracranial volume and pressure in patients with severe head injuries. Following upper abdominal or thoracic surgery or trauma, poor pain control may prevent the patient from coughing or breathing adequately and ventilation will allow paralysis, sedation and analgesia if indicated (Table 10.1).

The decision to initiate mechanical ventilation is based on clinical examination and arterial blood gas and metabolic abnormalities. Ventilation is usually necessary in a patient with one or more of the following: a $PaO_2 < 8\,kPa$ on maximal oxygen supplementation, high and increasing $PaCO_2$ values, acute respiratory acidosis or cardiovascular instability. Ventilation is also indicated for severe respiratory distress.[4] Arterial blood gases may not be grossly abnormal, but respiratory distress is manifested by a high respiratory rate (e.g. >30), low tidal volumes (e.g. <4 mL/kg), a low vital capacity (e.g. <15 mL/kg), along with symptoms of respiratory distress.

TABLE 10.1. Indications for mechanical ventilation

Failure to ventilate		
• Neurological	Central	Depressed ventilatory drive from intracerebral pathology (e.g. CVA), alcohol and other sedative or narcotic medication
	Spinal	Cervical and high thoracic spinal cord injury
	Peripheral	Guillain-Barré, polio, motor neurone disease, paralysing drugs, tetanus
• Muscle	Myopathies	Myasthenia, protein malnutrition
• Anatomical	Chest wall	Rib fractures, flail chest, chest wall deformities (e.g. scoliosis), morbid obesity, ascites, abdominal distension, restrictive dressings
	Pleura	Effusions, pneumothorax, haemothorax
	Airways	Obstruction (in lumen, in wall, outside wall), small tracheal tube, laryngeal oedema, foreign body, bronchospasm
Failure of gas exchange		
	Diffusion	Pulmonary oedema, ARDS, fibrosis, pneumonia
	Dead space	Pulmonary embolism, emphysema, cystic fibrosis, excessive PEEP
	Shunt	Lung collapse, atelectasis, consolidation
Other indications		To decrease oxygen consumption
		To control intracranial pressure
		To allow paralysis, sedation and analgesia

Intubation

Patients may be intubated because of upper airway obstruction, to protect the airway or facilitate control of secretions. In healthy adults there is little additional work of breathing with minute ventilation of less than 10 L/min through a tracheal tube of 7 mm or larger. Modes of spontaneous and supported ventilation incorporating positive end-expiratory pressure may be acceptable in some of these patients. However, many critically ill patients require higher minute ventilation, are weak and are cardiovascularly compromised and will require controlled ventilatory support.

Non-invasive Positive Pressure Ventilation

NIPPV avoids the need for intubation. It is most commonly indicated for managing acute exacerbations of chronic obstructive pulmonary disease (COPD) and to facilitate weaning from prolonged ventilation.[5,6] It may be suitable for many other situations; these include acute cardiogenic pulmonary oedema, avoidance of intubation in immunocompromised patients, asthma, postoperative respiratory failure, profound muscle weakness and chest wall deformity. NIPPV may also be considered in patients who have declined intubation or where this intervention is not thought to be appropriate.

Ventilatory Support in Specific Conditions

Acute Exacerbation of COPD

Suggested criteria for non-invasive and invasive ventilation are outlined in Table 10.2. Decisions about ventilation are guided by clinical experience and the response of the patient over time. In particular, if the patient remains conscious and cooperative, a trial of NIPPV may be justified even with a low pH, high PaCO$_2$ and low PaO$_2$.

Neuromuscular Disease

This includes conditions such as Guillain-Barré and Myasthenia Gravis. Vital capacity of less than 10–15 mL/kg and maximum inspiratory pressure of less than 20–30 cmH$_2$O have been suggested as

TABLE 10.2. Suggested criteria for ventilation in COPD

Non-invasive—at least two of the following
- Moderate to severe dyspnoea with use of accessory muscles
- Moderate acidosis (pH 7.3–7.35)
- Hypercapnia (PaCO$_2$ 6–8 kPa)
- Poor oxygenation (PaO$_2$/FiO$_2$ < 25 kPa)
- Respiratory rate > 25 breaths/min

Invasive ventilation–any of the following
- Severe dyspnoea with use of accessory muscles
- Severe acidosis (pH < 7.25)
- Hypercapnia (PaCO$_2$ > 8 kPa)
- Severe refractory hypoxaemia (PaO$_2$/FiO$_2$ < 10 kPa)
- Respiratory rate > 35 breaths/min
- Respiratory arrest
- Coma (GCS ≤ 8)
- Cardiovascular instability or other major complications
- High risk of aspiration
- Contraindications/limitations to NIPPV—e.g. morbid obesity, craniofacial trauma, recent upper airway or gastrointestinal surgery

indications for positive pressure ventilation. However, even below these thresholds ventilation may be manageable with non-invasive techniques in patients who can protect their airways. These techniques include NIPPV and negative pressure cuirass ventilation, either continuously or intermittently, in combination with physiotherapy and equipment to assist coughing and mobilisation of secretions.

Heart Failure and Cardiogenic Shock

Ventilation is hypothesised to decrease oxygen consumption at the time of severely reduced cardiac output. There is limited evidence from animal and patient studies to suggest that this may be beneficial.

Head Injury

Control of PaCO$_2$ affects cerebral blood flow and volume and it is important when managing a patient with severe intracranial injury. There are other indications for ventilation in these circumstances including avoidance of hypoxia and protection of the airway.

Flail Chest

Although intubation and ventilation used to be routine for patients with a flail chest, it is often unnecessary if the underlying lung function is adequate and appropriate analgesia is delivered allowing the patient to breathe and cough without pain.

High-Frequency Ventilation

High-frequency oscillatory and percussive ventilation have been tried in many circumstances including severe lung damage, inhalation injury and bronchopleural fistula.[7–11] This mode of ventilation may improve gas exchange while providing adequate ventilation at lower peak pressures than conventional ventilation. There may therefore be less risk of ventilator-induced lung injury.

Negative Pressure Ventilation

NPV is delivered through a cuirass ventilator such as an iron lung[12] or Hayek Oscillator.[13,14] Studies have shown that this form of ventilation can be effective in COPD and other forms of acute respiratory failure. Cardiac function may be better preserved with NPV than positive pressure ventilation.[15] Continuous negative external pressure may also improve cardiac as well as respiratory function.

Hazards of Mechanical Ventilation

Although in some circumstances intubation and ventilation is undoubtedly life-saving it is also associated with many risks and complications including pneumothorax, ventilator-associated pneumonia and ventilator-induced lung injury.[16,17] There are also additional hazards associated with the procedure of intubation itself, perhaps the most worrying being failure to intubate the trachea with the associated risk of hypoxic neurological damage. In patients ventilated for more than a brief time, outcomes are improved using 'lung protective' strategies to limit lung distension and transalveolar pressure.[18] Ventilation is also expensive and may be uncomfortable in the awake patient. There are few major complications associated with NIPPV but minor complications include nasal bridge ulceration, facial ulceration, epistaxis, increased intraocular pressure, gastric distension and aspiration, and poor tolerance/compliance.

References

1. Badar T, Bidani A. Mechanical ventilatory support. *Chest Surg Clin North Am.* 2002;12:265–299.

2. Pierson DJ. Indications for mechanical ventilation in adults with acute respiratory failure. *Respir Care.* 2002;47:249–262.

3. Sevransky JE, Levy MM, Marini JJ. Mechanical ventilation in sepsis-induced acute lung injury/acute respiratory distress syndrome: an evidence-based review. *Crit Care Med.* 2004;32:S548–S553.

4. Rabinstein AA, Wijdicks EF. Warning signs of imminent respiratory failure in neurological patients. *Semin Neurol.* 2003;23:97–104.

5. Liesching T, Kwok H, Hill NS. Acute applications of noninvasive positive pressure ventilation. *Chest.* 2003;124:699–713.

6. Shneerson JM, Simonds AK. Noninvasive ventilation for chest wall and neuromuscular disorders. *Eur Respir J.* 2002;20:480–487.

7. Cartotto R, Ellis S, Smith T. Use of high-frequency oscillatory ventilation in burn patients. *Crit Care Med.* 2005;33:S175–S181.

8. Chan KP, Stewart TE. Clinical use of high-frequency oscillatory ventilation in adult patients with acute respiratory distress syndrome. *Crit Care Med.* 2005;33:S170–S174.

9. Derdak S. High-frequency oscillatory ventilation for adult acute respiratory distress syndrome: a decade of progress. *Crit Care Med.* 2005;33:S113–S114.

10. Imai Y, Slutsky AS. High-frequency oscillatory ventilation and ventilator-induced lung injury. *Crit Care Med.* 2005;33:S129–S134.

11. Salim A, Martin M. High-frequency percussive ventilation. *Crit Care Med.* 2005;33:S241–S245.

12. Corrado A, Ginanni R, Villella G, Gorini M, Augustynen A, Tozzi D, et al. Iron lung versus conventional mechanical ventilation in acute exacerbation of COPD. *Eur Respir J.* 2004;23:419–424.

13. Al Saady NM, Fernando SS, Petros AJ, Cummin AR, Sidhu VS, Bennett ED. External high frequency oscillation in normal subjects and in patients with acute respiratory failure. *Anaesthesia.* 1995;50:1031–1035.

14. Sideno B, Vaage J. Ventilation by external high-frequency oscillations improves cardiac function after coronary artery bypass grafting. *Eur J Cardiothorac Surg.* 1997;11:248–257.

15. Torelli L, Zoccali G, Casarin, Dalla Zuanna F, Lieta E, Conti G. Comparative evaluation of the haemodynamic effects of continuous negative external pressure (CNEP) and positive end-expiratory pressure (PEEP) in mechanically ventilated trauma patients. *Intensive Care Med.* 1995;21:67–70.

16. Ferguson ND, Frutos-Vivar F, Esteban A, Anzueto A, Alía I, Brower RG, et al. Airway pressures, tidal volumes, and mortality in patients with acute respiratory distress syndrome. *Crit Care Med.* 2005;33:21–30.

17. Gajic O, Frutos-Vivar F, Esteban, Hubmayr RD, Anzueto A. Ventilator settings as a risk factor for acute respiratory distress syndrome in mechanically ventilated patients. *Intensive Care Med.* 2005; 31:922–926.

18. Moran JL, Bersten AD, Solomon PJ. Meta-analysis of controlled trials of ventilator therapy in acute lung injury and acute respiratory distress syndrome: an alternative perspective. *Intensive Care Med.* 2005;31:227–235.

11
Modes of Invasive and Non-invasive Ventilatory Support

Tony Pickworth

Abstract The respiratory system is susceptible to insults from many sources, both intra- and extra-pulmonary, and is the organ system supported most frequently in critically ill patients. In broad terms, the need for respiratory support may arise due to a failure of ventilation or oxygenation. Although institution of mechanical ventilation can be life-saving in these circumstances, it may also lead to ventilator-induced lung injury (VILI) through barotrauma, volutrauma and oxygen toxicity, and strategies to minimise VILI must be incorporated within the overall approach.

Developing a consistent approach to mechanical ventilation is made more complex by the myriad of acronyms and trademarked names used by the different equipment manufacturers. These serve to confuse by means of having very similar functions and names. In fact there is little evidence for the superiority of one mode of ventilation over another. The aim of this chapter is to explain the basic principles on which these systems are based, and enable the reader to build a sound strategy for delivering respiratory support to critically ill patients.

Abbreviations

APRV	Airway pressure release ventilation
ARDS	Acute respiratory distress syndrome
BIPAP	Biphasic positive airway pressure
BiPAP™	Bilevel positive airway pressure
COPD	Chronic obstructive pulmonary disease
CPAP	Continuous positive airway pressure
T_{exp}	Expiratory time
ECMO	Extra corporeal membrane oxygenation
FiO_2	Inspired fraction of oxygen
Q	Inspiratory flow rate
T_{insp}	Inspiratory time
T_{ir}	Inspiratory rise time
T_p	Inspiratory pause time
P_{insp}	Inspiratory pressure
IPPB	Intermittent positive pressure breathing
IRV	Inverse ratio ventilation
MV	Minute volume
P_{max}	Maximum pressure
NIPPV	Non-invasive positive pressure ventilation
P_{supp}	Pressure support
PEEP	Positive end expiratory pressure
PRVC	Pressure-regulated volume control
SIMV	Synchronised intermittent mandatory ventilation
VC	Volume control
VA-ECMO	Veno-arterial ECMO
VV-ECMO	Veno-venous ECMO

Introduction

Mechanical respiratory support can be subdivided into three categories:

- Mechanical support without ventilation
- Negative pressure ventilation
- Positive pressure ventilation.

In these systems 'negative' is taken to mean pressure less than atmospheric and 'positive' more than atmospheric.

Respiratory Support Without Ventilation

The most basic mechanical intervention used in critically ill patients is continuous positive airway pressure (CPAP). This is sometimes referred to as continuous positive pressure breathing (CPPB), and was first used in the 1930s to treat pulmonary oedema.[1] Essentially it requires a system that can maintain a constant positive pressure which varies by no more than $2–3\,cmH_2O$ over the respiratory cycle. In order to prevent pressure falling during inspiration a high flow of gas must be applied to the system. There has to be a mechanism for preventing rebreathing and an expiratory valve that sets the nominal CPAP level. This offers no ventilatory support, but enhances oxygenation through increasing mean airway pressure.

A number of CPAP systems have developed over time but two types are particularly prevalent:

- *Reservoir bag systems.* These use a gas reservoir to provide adequate gas flow at the peak of inspiration. These systems also require an additional low-resistance one-way valve in the inspiratory limb to prevent rebreathing. This type would include the Drager CF800 system (Figure 11.1).
- *Air entrainment systems* such as the Whispa Flow. These use the Venturi principle to entrain air into an oxygen delivery system. High gas flows are delivered to the patient, so the pressure drop is minimal during the peak of inspiration. The high flow also ensures that rebreathing of expired gas is prevented.

The expiratory valves are usually spring-loaded systems which operate at low preset pressures (Figure 11.2).

Intermittent Negative Pressure Ventilation

Application of an intermittent negative pressure to the chest wall may improve ventilation in some groups of patients. 'Iron lungs' are intermittent negative pressure tank ventilators that enclose the entire body, apart from the head, and can provide complete ventilatory support to patients with abnormalities of the chest wall. However, they cannot generate sufficient pressure differences to support patients with severely impaired lung function. Cuirass or jacket ventilators deliver partial support, but their performance is often limited by leaks, and they are often associated with the development of pressure sores.

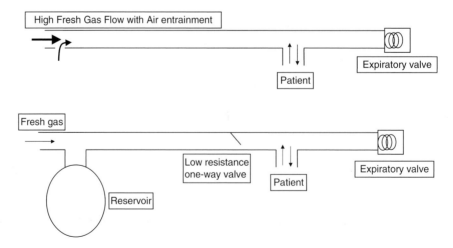

FIGURE 11.1. Two systems for delivering continuous positive airway pressure (CPAP). The first uses a reservoir bag to provide adequate gas flow to the patient during inspiration and a one-way inspiratory valve to prevent rebreathing. The second uses air entrainment to generate a high enough flow. An inspiratory valve is not required to prevent rebreathing. The simple and successful Boussignac system essentially works on this principle.

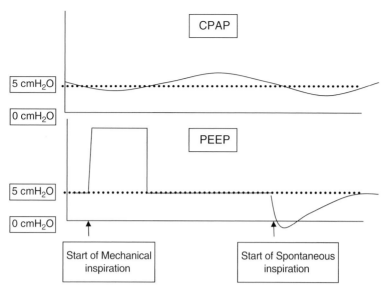

FIGURE 11.2. What is the difference between CPAP and PEEP? Positive end-expiratory pressure (PEEP) is the application of a positive pressure (above atmospheric) to the airway during expiration, usually by means of an expiratory valve. Unlike CPAP, where the pressure must be maintained throughout the entire respiratory cycle, PEEP only requires the pressure to be maintained during expiration. A high gas flow is therefore not needed. The effect of PEEP on gas exchange is similar to that of CPAP. PEEP is usually employed in conjunction with intermittent positive pressure ventilation, during which a positive pressure is maintained throughout the cycle. However, if the patient attempts to breathe spontaneously, the respiratory effort may generate sub-atmospheric pressures during the spontaneous inspiratory phase.

Intermittent Positive Pressure Ventilation

Basic Modes of Ventilation

The most common modes of ventilation can be described by the way in which the ventilator delivers a breath of a certain magnitude, and the way in which it cycles between expiration and inspiration. A breath can be delivered as volume preset or pressure preset. The cycling can be determined by the patient (a supported breath) or the ventilator (a controlled breath). Based on this assumption a simple matrix generates four potential modes of ventilation.

	Controlled	Supported
Volume preset	Volume control	Volume support
Pressure preset	Pressure control	Pressure support

To make things simpler, volume support is not a widely used mode, so we will ignore it here and consider only three modes: volume control, pressure control and pressure support.

Volume Control

Volume control delivers a set tidal volume (determined by the operator) at regular time intervals (again set by the operator) to the patient. In order to do this, the following parameters should be set on the ventilator:

- Tidal volume (V_T)
- Inspiratory flow rate (Q)
- Total inspiratory time (T_{insp})
- Frequency (f)

These four parameters are important because they describe the 'breath shape', and this will influence the effectiveness of the breath in terms of lung recruitment (Figure 11.3). From these four basic parameters others can be derived. The settings on many ventilators will use some of these derived parameters. This is because of historical user familiarity with the concepts encompassed by the derived parameters. Derived parameters include:

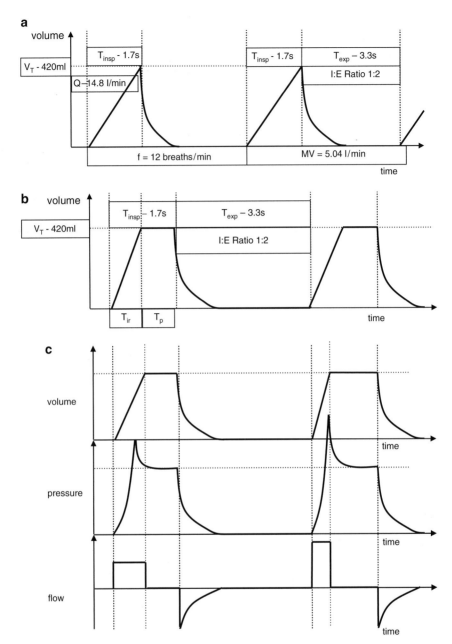

Figure 11.3. ((a) The four parameters V_T, T_{insp}, f and Q (the gradient of the slope) define the shape of the breath. These are shown in the first breath. Note the flow of 14.8 L/min (or 247 mL/s) means that a V_T of 420 mL can be delivered in 1.7 s. The second breath shows how other parameters are derived. At a respiratory frequency of 12 each breath is 5 s in duration so T_{exp} is 3.3 s (5–1.7 s). Therefore, the I/E ratio is 1:2. The MV is 5.04 l (420 mL × 12). (b) The flow rate has been increased leading to development of a pause time. However the total inspiratory time remains unchanged, as does the I/E ratio. (c) The volume pressure and flow curves are shown as contemporaneous. Note the overshoot in the pressure curve that settles to a plateau once flow ceases. The second breath is delivered with a higher flow rate. This generates a higher mean airway volume but at the expense of a marked increase in airway pressure.

- Minute volume (MV) [$V_T \times f$]
- Inspiratory rise time (T_{ir}) [V_T/Q]
- Pause time (T_p) [$T_{insp} - T_{ir}$]
- Expiratory time (T_{exp}) [$60/f - T_{insp}$],
- I/E ratio [T_{insp}/T_{exp}].

By using these derived parameters to set the ventilator the breath shape can still be determined. Adjusting the settings leads to changes in breath shape which may be advantageous in terms of ventilatory strategy. For example, if the flow rate is increased then the tidal volume is achieved earlier. For a constant T_{insp} a pause time T_p is introduced. During this time there is no flow of gas into or out of the lungs. The greater the flow rate the earlier V_T is achieved. This leads to a greater mean airway volume which leads to an improvement in lung recruitment and oxygenation.

As gas flow increases, airway resistance also rises generating higher airway pressures. It has been argued that this pressure is dissipated by the time the gas reaches the alveoli. However in patients with severe lung disease different alveoli are likely to have different time constants, hence the pressure may be dissipated unevenly through-out the lung and a large overshoot may result in lung damage or barotrauma. The differing time constants may also lead to movement of gas between lung units, termed *pendelluft*.

Pressure Control

The optimum compromise between high flow and low pressure is delivered by pressure control ventilation. The operator sets the inspiratory pressure (P_{insp}), thus protecting the lung from extremes of pressure, with flow being determined by the time constant of the lung.

When setting the ventilator in pressure control mode, three basic parameters are adjusted:

- Inspiratory pressure (P_{insp})
- Total inspiratory time (T_{insp})
- Frequency (f)

During the early part of a breath gas flow is fast, due to the large pressure difference between the ventilator circuit and the lungs, and lung volume increases rapidly. Gas flow then decelerates as the ventilator and lungs equilibrate. At this point there may be an inspiratory pause (Figure 11.4).

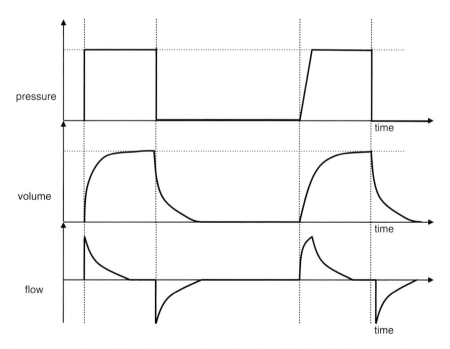

FIGURE 11.4. Pressure control breaths deliver the optimum breath shape. The tidal volume is dependent on lung compliance, but is delivered quickly without sharp rises in pressure. The rate of pressure change from expiration to inspiration can also be changed as in the second breath. This is often referred to as the ramp.

The I:E ratio is determined by T_{insp} and f as for volume control. The tidal volume and hence minute volume are dependent on the lung mechanics. The main disadvantage of pressure control ventilation is that the tidal volume may fall if the lungs become stiff, or may increase as lung mechanics improve. High tidal volumes (12 mL/kg ideal body weight) are associated with worse outcome and must therefore be avoided.

One other ventilator setting is applicable on some machines. This is the 'ramp' or rate of change of pressure from expiration to inspiration. The ramp time is usually very short (around 0.2 s). It is rarely necessary to adjust the ramp in pressure control mode.

Pressure Support

Pressure support (sometimes referred to as assisted spontaneous breathing [ASB]) is a common mode of ventilation for patients who have reasonably well-preserved respiratory control mechanisms. The magnitude of support is determined by a preset inspiratory pressure but the cycling from expiration to inspiration and back is determined by patient factors (Figure 11.5). The only settings required are positive end-expiratory pressure (PEEP) and pressure support level which we will call P_{supp} (Box 11.1).

Cycling from expiration to inspiration (triggering of the ventilator) is initiated by the patient's own respiratory effort. The ventilator then generates an inspiratory pressure as set by P_{supp}. Early versions employed a pressure trigger but modern ventilators use a flow trigger which requires less work to operate (Box 11.2).

For cycling from inspiration to expiration most ventilators work on an algorithm, for example, when flow rate falls to a fixed percentage (usually between 5% and 25%) of the maximum flow generated during the breath. Note that, unlike the controlled modes of ventilation, if the patient makes no respiratory effort there will be no ventilation.

The only other variable is the 'ramp', which may require adjustment in certain circumstances. If an excessively fast rate of change is applied inspiratory muscle activity may be suppressed, and the patient effectively allows the ventilator to do the work. Conversely if a very low rate of change is applied, the patient makes continued effort against limited airflow. This increases the work of breathing and may result in respiratory failure.

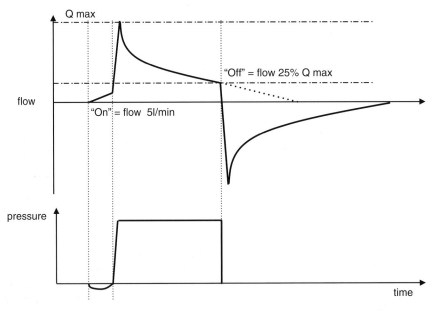

FIGURE 11.5. Pressure Support. The breath is triggered 'on' by spontaneous effort. Detection of inward flow of gas leads to cycling to the inspiratory pressure (preset). As a pressure breath the flow has a decelerating waveform just as one sees in pressure control. There is a peak flow rate shortly after the inspiratory pressure has been reached. The flow decreases. In this instance the ventilator cycles to expiration when the flow rate has fallen to 25% of its maximum.

Box 11.1. Potential pitfalls—pressure settings

A potential pitfall is that on many ventilators P_{insp} for pressure control is an absolute value whereas P_{supp} for pressure support may be set as 'above PEEP'. This can lead to misunderstandings as to what is set on the ventilator especially as these two modes can be employed at the same time. So with PEEP set to 10 cmH$_2$O a P_{insp} of 15 cmH$_2$O will lead to a pressure difference of 5 cmH$_2$O and a peak pressure of 15 cmH$_2$O, whereas a P_{supp} of 15 cmH$_2$O may be 'above PEEP' in which case the peak pressure will be 25 cmH$_2$O.

Box 11.2. Triggering ventilators

Early versions of pressure support utilised a pressure trigger. When the patient caused the circuit pressure to fall to a preset level (usually 2–3 cmH$_2$O below expiratory pressure) then the ventilator would cycle to inspiration. This often required more work than might be anticipated as the compliance of the breathing circuit would absorb some of the pressure change. Modern ventilators operate a flow trigger whereby during expiration there is a constant flow of gas through the circuit out of the expiratory valve. The ventilator can detect any change in flow rate without the need to alter pressure significantly. This makes it easier to trigger.

There is a slight catch though….

Many patients will experience what is known as intrinsic PEEP. This is where the pressure in the lung at end expiration remains above the circuit pressure, often as a result of limitation of expiratory airflow. In this case patients will have to overcome intrinsic PEEP in order to equilibrate with the circuit pressure before they can start to generate flow into the lung and trigger the ventilator. This can lead to increased work of breathing and respiratory failure. The remedy is to match extrinsic PEEP (i.e. that set on the ventilator) to intrinsic PEEP. That way the circuit pressure and lung pressure are the same and any additional effort allows flow of gas and triggering occurs.

Dual Modes of Ventilation (Pressure-Regulated Volume Control)

From an oxygenation perspective pressure control ventilation delivers the optimal 'breath shape', and is commonly used when patients have severe oxygenation failure. However with pressure control there is a risk, particularly if lung compliance improves, that excessively high tidal volumes may be inadvertently delivered resulting in lung damage. To address this problem 'dual modes' have been developed that incorporate elements of both volume and pressure control.

As demonstrated in Figure 11.3c, if high inspiratory flows are used excessive pressure may be applied to the lung. This can be avoided by applying a pressure regulator to the inspiratory phase, to prevent occurrence of high peaks, while instructing the ventilator to deliver a high inspiratory flow to

maximise mean airway pressure and lung recruitment (Figure 11.6). This is the most basic form of pressure-regulated volume control (PRVC). In this form V_T can be set to 6 mL/kg, and inspiratory flow

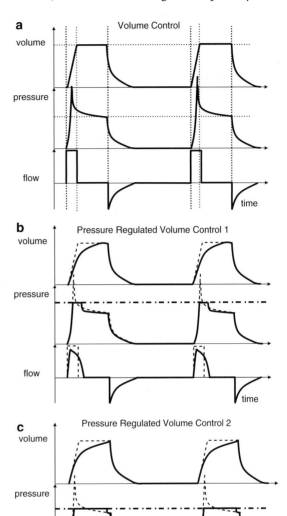

Figure 11.6. (a) In the first diagram we see the effect of application of high inspiratory flow rate on peak airway pressure.
(b) If we start to regulate maximum pressure the flow rate becomes limited and as we further regulate the pressure the breath shape takes on the *form* of a pressure control breath.
(c) It is not possible to further limit the inspiratory pressure as the lung compliance here would not permit the delivery of the set tidal volume within these parameters.

rate to a nominal maximum (e.g. 120 L/min). A pressure maximum (P_{max}) can be set and adjusted to 2 or 3 cmH$_2$O above that required to allow the ventilator to deliver the full tidal volume.

Most commercial forms of PRVC simplify things further. A preset V_T is entered but there is no flow setting or maximum pressure setting. For a number of initial breaths a constant, low flow, volume-controlled breath is delivered and the peak pressure measured. This gives an idea of lung compliance from which the ventilator can determine the P_{insp} required to deliver the preset V_T. The measurement of V_T allows the ventilator to assess whether for the subsequent breath the inspiratory pressure (P_{insp}) should be higher, lower or the same. Using this system the ventilator maintains V_T for the lowest inspiratory pressure. This system is described as Autoflow™ by Drager and may be used in volume control modes with their EVITA series of ventilators. However, it should be noted that most ventilators offering PRVC also operate in this way.

PRVC has advantages in offering the optimal breath shape seen with pressure control while allowing predetermination of the V_T.[2] It is also quite simple to set, requiring only three parameters. However, in patients with a high respiratory drive PRVC can be problematic. If the patient breathes during the inspiratory cycle then the V_T increases. The ventilator then makes a downward adjustment to the P_{insp} as it is confused into thinking lung compliance has improved. As the pressure decreases more effort takes place and the ventilator can be fooled into delivering less and less inspiratory pressure until it is almost zero. While in some circumstances it might be appropriate for this 'auto-weaning' to occur, for patients with severe oxygenation failure this can lead to inappropriately increased work of breathing and some de-recruitment of lung units.

Add-Ons and Modifications

Although most modes of mechanical ventilation can be fitted into the matrix described (i.e. volume control, pressure control or pressure support), there are also a number of complementary systems, which have been developed to either promote weaning from the ventilator or to enhance oxygenation.

Synchronised Intermittent Mandatory Ventilation (SIMV)

SIMV is a very commonly employed system. The concept itself is simple and designed to facilitate some spontaneous breathing during mechanical ventilation. In early ICU ventilators the delivery of breaths was mandatory (MV), and the patient could not initiate or effect any spontaneous breaths. By inserting a valve into the expiratory limb of the ventilator circuit, patients were also able to take spontaneous breaths. This arrangement was termed intermittent mandatory ventilation (IMV),[3] and IMV valves were often used when weaning commenced. However, this system had a number of disadvantages, including delivery of an excessive tidal volume to the patient if a spontaneous breath was taken just prior to a mandatory one. The resulting rise in airway pressure would usually trigger a pressure alarm, and the breath could be 'cut-off'. High airway pressures could also be generated as the patient tried to exhale.

In extreme cases this patient–ventilator asynchrony ('patient fighting the ventilator') might result in ventilatory failure.

Using the same triggering systems employed in pressure support, it is now possible to synchronise spontaneous and mandatory breaths. If the patient triggers the ventilator within a certain time window before a breath is due, then the mandatory breath can be initiated early. Different ventilators have different trigger windows. Usually triggering can occur within the last 25% or so of the expiratory phase. This can lead to the delivery of more mandatory breaths than prescribed and different ventilators have specific strategies to cope with this. Either more breaths are permitted or compensatory lengthening of the subsequent expiratory phase is allowed.

SIMV is therefore only a timing/triggering system and not a mode of ventilation in its own right. It can be applied to volume-control (VC-SIMV), pressure-control (PC-SIMV) or indeed PRVC (PRVC-SIMV). SIMV was designed to facilitate weaning. As spontaneous effort increased, the frequency of mandatory ventilation could be reduced until full spontaneous ventilation was achieved. The spontaneous ventilation could also be supported using pressure support, and one of the commonest systems of mechanical ventilation is

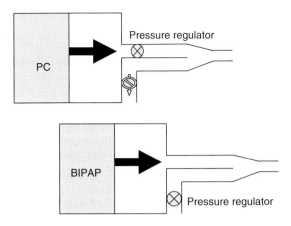

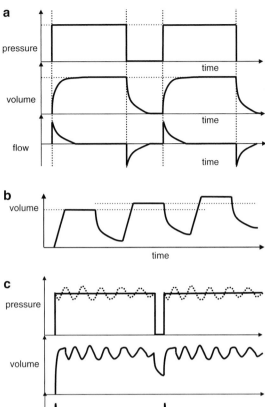

FIGURE 11.7. Pressure control differs from BIPAP only in the position of the pressure regulator. In PC this is part of the inspiratory valve whereas in BIPAP it is part of the expiratory valve.

SIMV + pressure support. Although this system of weaning was employed for many years, randomised controlled trials have demonstrated that SIMV weaning is actually less effective than either pressure support weaning or simple T-piece weaning. Nevertheless, SIMV systems may still have a role in encouraging some spontaneous breathing when active weaning is not being undertaken, and in helping to reduce patient–ventilator asynchrony.

Biphasic Positive Airway Pressure (BIPAP)

This is a relatively new development in the realm of pressure control ventilation, and often causes some confusion due to the existence of many almost identical modes with similar trademarked names and acronyms.[4,5] Technically the development is simple. In many ventilators breaths are delivered via inspiratory and expiratory valves. In pressure control during inspiration the pressure delivered (P_{insp}) is generated from the inspiratory end of the circuit while the expiratory valve is closed. During expiration the inspiratory valve is closed and the expiratory valve opens to allow exhalation. The expiratory valve may also permit the delivery of positive end-expiratory pressure (PEEP) (Figure 11.7). In BIPAP the expiratory valve becomes a pressure valve which switches between P_{insp} and PEEP. Essentially there is no inspiratory valve but there is a constant high gas flow through the circuit. Pressure cycles between

FIGURE 11.8. (a) Inverse ratio ventilation utilised here in pressure control mode. The area under the pressure and volume curves are much increased compared to the original pressure control curves in Figure 11.4. However the peak pressure and tidal volume are unchanged. This manoeuvre will increase oxygenation by improving lung recruitment. (b) Breath stacking. When there is inadequate time for full expiration breath stacking may occur. Therefore the lung volume has not fallen to its original level. In volume control ventilation an additional tidal volume is delivered so the lung volume for each subsequent breath increases. This leads to increasing peak airway pressures and may trigger an alarm. As the peak pressure rises the expiratory flow rate will increase so this may not be an inexorable rise and a new stable state may be achieved. If pressure control ventilation is used we don't consider the result to be breath stacking, but what happens is similar. The intrinsic PEEP increases while the P_{insp} remains the same so V_T falls. (c) Airway pressure release ventilation (APRV). The patient generates small, rapid breaths at a high pressure. Carbon dioxide elimination is enhanced by brief periods of reduced pressure that are equivalent to very short expiratory times.

P_{insp} and PEEP in both PC and BIPAP, so that ventilation occurs as the pressure in the lungs changes to equilibrate with the ventilator.

To understand the benefits of the BIPAP system, it is helpful to consider a patient who tries to take a spontaneous breath during the ventilator inspiratory cycle. By generating spontaneous effort the pressure in the lungs falls so gas moves from ventilator to patient and both BIPAP and PC allow the ventilator to replenish that gas in order to maintain the set pressure. However, in pressure control ventilation a problem occurs when the patient then tries to exhale. The expiratory valve remains closed, and since gas cannot pass back through the inspiratory valve, a high pressure is generated which triggers the ventilator alarms and cuts the breath off. Under these circumstances patient–ventilator asynchrony occurs and inadequate ventilation may be observed. In BIPAP, in order to exhale during the inspiratory phase the patient only has to generate a higher pressure than the P_{insp} and gas will flow out through the expiratory valve. The breath is not lost and asynchrony does not usually occur. Under normal circumstances it is unusual for a patient to attempt to breathe during a mandatory inspiration; however, it does become an issue when a long T_{insp} is used, especially if the patient has a raised arterial carbon dioxide tension and high respiratory drive. Hence in patients with severe lung disease in whom long inspiratory times are being used, it is often necessary to administer neuromuscular blocking agents to facilitate effective pressure control ventilation. This is rarely necessary when using BIPAP. Apart from this technical advantage, the settings and breath delivery are the same for both modes.

Ventilatory Strategies to Enhance Oxygenation

When oxygenation remains a problem despite instigation of mechanical ventilation measures should be taken to increase mean airway pressure. Since this must be done without exceeding safe peak pressures or tidal volumes, the options are to increase PEEP or T_{insp}.

Inverse Ratio Ventilation

If the frequency is unchanged but T_{insp} is increased, then the I/E ratio will alter from its usual 1:2 to 2:1 (e.g. f 12, T_{insp} 3.4 s, T_{exp} 1.7 s). This is known as inverse ratio ventilation (IRV)[6] (Figure 11.8a). The reduction of T_{exp} and increase in functional residual capacity of the lung in relation to tidal volume leads towards hypercapnoea, which in turn results in increased respiratory drive. IRV may be less successful using volume control because if T_{exp} is inadequate it may lead to 'breath stacking' (Figure 11.8b). IRV is more usually applied with pressure control, which gives rise to the acronym PC-IRV.

Positive End-Expiratory Pressure (PEEP)

Application of PEEP can recruit lung tissue by increasing mean airway pressure, in the same way that CPAP does for patients breathing spontaneously.[7] Like CPAP it does not contribute to 'ventilation' but does help oxygenation. Much debate has been generated about how much PEEP is appropriate to apply. Increased PEEP may lead to a decrease in cardiac output, and 'best PEEP' was often considered to be that which gave the best oxygen delivery. However, we now recognise the importance of PEEP in preventing repeated alveolar collapse at end expiration as part of a lung-protective ventilatory strategy, and levels high enough to open the lung and keep it open should be used wherever possible.

Strategies for Severe Oxygenation Failure

Airway Pressure Release Ventilation (APRV)

Normally IRV is considered as a 2:1 or maximally 3:1 ratio. With the development of BIPAP this can be extended such that the expiratory times are very small and the ratio can be of the order of 9:1. As the patient can breathe during the inspiratory part of the cycle there is often fast, low V_T, spontaneous respiration during the inspiratory phase. In essence this is high level CPAP, with brief periods (0.5 s) of enhanced expiration, which helps to eliminate CO_2 and is known as airway pressure release ventilation or APRV.[8] This has been shown to be a safe and effective mode of ventilation in severe ARDS.

High Frequency Oscillation

The theoretical end to this strategy is infinite I/E ratio or lung inflation but no ventilation. This strategy would fail because of the inability to eliminate CO_2, which would lead to severe acidosis and falling alveolar oxygen concentration. CO_2 would diffuse out of the lung along the bronchial tree down a concentration gradient as long as the airway is open but not fast enough to prevent hypoxia and severe acidosis. However, if oscillation is applied to the airway, this facilitates diffusion of CO_2 out of the alveoli at a rate that permits adequate gas exchange. Oscillators essentially are able to improve oxygenation by applying a relatively high mean airway pressure to the lung.[9] CO_2 clearance is achieved by a vibrating cone superimposing low-volume high-frequency (3–15 Hz) breaths around the mean airway pressure.

Extra-corporeal Membrane Oxygenation (ECMO)

In the event that adequate oxygenation cannot be achieved using the lungs, the blood can be oxygenated (and CO_2 removed) using an extracorporeal circuit.[10] ECMO circuits can be set up as veno-arterial circuits (VA-ECMO) when both cardiac and respiratory support is required or as veno-venous circuits (VV-ECMO) for respiratory support only. When ECMO is used some ventilation may be applied to the lung but usually at low rate and low tidal volume. The idea of this strategy is to reduce the ventilator-induced component of the lung injury and allow time for the lung to heal.

Non-invasive Mechanical Respiratory Support

Non-invasive CPAP for pulmonary oedema was described in the 1930s and non-invasive ventilatory support (IPPB) as an aid to physiotherapy using a bird ventilator was well described in the

---

Box 11.3. What's the difference between BIPAP and BiPAP™?

In both these systems two levels of CPAP are applied to the patient. Biphasic positive airway pressure (BIPAP) is a way of delivering pressure controlled ventilation. However, bilevel positive airway pressure (BiPAP™) is usually cycled from expiration to inspiration by patient effort—in other words a form of pressure support. Considerable work has gone into the algorithm for triggering using the BiPAP™ system. The exact details are unpublished, but involve identifying points on the flow volume loop that appear to signify the optimum times to cycle from expiration to inspiration and vice versa.

1970s. Despite this, non-invasive techniques of respiratory support were not widely used until the late 1980s.

Theoretically any mode of mechanical support can be applied non-invasively, but some are more successful than others. The commonly used techniques are non-invasive CPAP, or non-invasive forms of pressure support—now usually referred to as non-invasive positive pressure ventilation (NIPPV). The most widely used form of NIPPV is probably BiPAP™ or bilevel positive airway pressure. This is a specific system patented by Respironics for their non-invasive ventilators, and is distinct from BIPAP as described above although there are common features (Box 11.3).

CPAP is useful in the treatment of pulmonary oedema, obstructive sleep apnoea and chronic obstructive pulmonary disease (COPD). NIPPV is most effectively used for patients with ventilatory failure due to neuromuscular disease or COPD.[11]

Non-invasive ventilators have different characteristics to invasive ventilators, and must be able to provide a sufficient flow of gas to compensate for leaks. Their alarm settings are also modified to detect significant air leaks. Since they are designed primarily for patients with ventilatory rather than oxygenation failure, the mechanisms for controlling FiO_2 are less well defined. The other major consideration is the interface between the ventilator and the patient. Devices include nasal masks, full face masks, nasal plugs and hoods, all of which have relative advantages and disadvantages in terms of claustrophobia, fitting and leak.

Use of NIPPV has led to a reduction in the need for intubation and mortality for patients with COPD, and offers an alternative strategy when there are ethical dilemmas about intubation in patients with irreversible disease. It may also have a role in a subgroup of patients who have recently been weaned from invasive ventilation and extubated. It is less useful for patients with more severe disease or for conditions other than COPD.

A Strategy for Mechanical Support

With all of these (and more) options available it can be difficult to identify the best strategy for an individual patient. To a large extent the approach taken will be determined by whether the patient has predominately oxygenation or ventilatory failure. The particular strategies favoured in my own unit are detailed in the following sections.

Patients with Oxygenation Failure

1. Treat the underlying cause
2. Chest physiotherapy to enhance lung recruitment
3. In cases of pulmonary oedema or COPD you may try non-invasive CPAP
4. When progressing to invasive ventilation start on a volume control mode—preferably as a dual mode (PRVC or Autoflow™). Set V_T to 6 mL/kg (ideal body weight) and never change this setting[12]
5. For worsening oxygenation increase PEEP and T_{insp}. Permit hypercapnoea within reasonable limits. Adjust PEEP and T_{insp} in order to try and keep FiO_2 0.6 or less
6. When I/E ratio is reversed it may be necessary to switch to pressure control (preferably BIPAP)
7. If oxygenation is still a problem despite PC-IRV and PEEP >15 cmH₂O, you may need to employ an alternative strategy such as APRV, oscillation or consider ECMO
8. As the patient improves encourage spontaneous breathing using pressure support
9. Wean from the ventilator using reducing levels of pressure support or T-piece weaning

Patients with Ventilation Failure

1. Treat the underlying cause
2. In COPD if pH >7.25 try NIPPV such as BiPAP™

3. When progressing to invasive ventilation start on a volume control mode—preferably as a dual mode (PRVC or Autoflow™). Set V_T to 6 mL/kg (ideal body weight) and never change this setting
4. Ensure there is adequate T_{exp} to allow reasonably full exhalation
5. If breath stacking occurs switch to pressure control
6. When the patient improves encourage spontaneous breathing using pressure support
7. Wean from ventilator using pressure support or T-piece weaning

References

1. Barach AL, Martin J, Eckman M. Positive pressure respiration and its application to the treatment of acute pulmonary edema. *Ann Intern Med.* 1938; 12:754–795.
2. Guldager H, Nielsen SL, Peder C, Sorensen MB. A comparison of volume control and pressure-regulated volume control ventilation in acute respiratory failure. *Crit Care.* 1997;1:75–77.
3. Downs JB, Klein EF Jr, Desautels D, Modell JH, Kirby RR. Intermittent mandatory ventilation: a new approach to weaning patients from mechanical ventilators. *Chest.* 1973;64(3):331–335.
4. Hörmann Ch, Baum M, Putensen Ch, Mutz NJ, Benzer H. Biphasic positive airway pressure (BIPAP)—a new mode of ventilatory support. *Eur J Anaesthesiol.* 1994;11:37–42.
5. MacIntyre NR, Gropper C, Westfall T. Combining pressure-limiting and volume-cycling features in a patient- interactive mechanical breath. *Crit Care Med.* 1994; 22(2):353–357.
6. Marcy TW, Marini JJ. Inverse ratio ventilation in ARDS. Rationale implementation. *Chest.* 1991;100: 494–504.
7. Smith TC, Marini JJ. Impact of PEEP on lung mechanics and work of breathing in severe airflow obstruction. *J Appl Physiol.* 1988;65: 1488–1499.
8. Stock MC, Downs JB, Frolicher DA. Airway pressure release ventilation. *Crit Care Med.* 1987; 15(5):462–466.
9. Mehta S, Lapinsk S, Hallett DC, et al. Prospective trial of high-frequency oscillation in adults with acute respiratory distress syndrome. *Crit Care Med.* 2001;29(7):1360–1369.
10. Zapol WM, Snider MT, Hill JD, et al. Extracorporeal membrane oxygenation in severe acute respiratory failure. *JAMA.* 1979;242:2193–2196.

11. Plant P, Owen J, Elliott M. Early use of non-invasive ventilation for acute exacerbations of chronic obstructive pulmonary disease on general respiratory wards: a multicentre randomised controlled trial. *The Lancet*. 2000;355:1931–1935.

12. The Acute Respiratory Distress Syndrome Network. Ventilation with lower tidal volumes as compared with traditional tidal volumes for acute lung injury and the acute respiratory distress syndrome. *NEJM*. 2000;342:1301–1308.

12
Blood Gas Measurement and Interpretation

Adrian J. Williams

Abstract Arterial blood gas (ABG) measurements commonly guide therapy in Intensive Care and High Dependency Units and require a full understanding for accurate interpretation. Robust electrodes provide precise values for pH, $PaCO_2$ and PaO_2 and calculated values of HCO_3^-, base excess and anion gap are extremely useful. From these, it is possible to identify and describe any disturbance in acid–base status. Hypoxaemia due to lung pathology can be distinguished from pure hypoventilation through calculation of the alveolar–arterial oxygen gradient. A clinical approach to the systematic assessment of arterial blood gas measurements is suggested and controversies relating to temperature correction, suitability of capillary samples and pulse oximetry are discussed.

Introduction

The measurement of arterial pH, PCO_2 and PO_2, more commonly referred to as arterial blood gases (ABGs), is ubiquitous in medical practice. They are often the most precise measurements which, with careful and methodical interpretation, can successfully guide therapy. A proper understanding of the pathophysiology behind the measurements, their rapid interpretation and an appreciation of their limitations is essential in the critical care environment. In this chapter, I offer a personal view, gleaned and honed during more than 40 years of practice and teaching.

Why are ABGs done? Although levels of oxygenation can be approximated with pulse oximetry, ABGs are frequently taken to quantify *oxygenation* and guide oxygen therapy. Calculation of the *alveolar–arterial oxygen gradient* may provide evidence for or against lung disease and suggest a pathophysiological process. The adequacy of *ventilation* can be assessed from the level of $PaCO_2$ ($PaCO_2 \propto {}^1\!/\text{ventilation}$). ABGs may also identify *acid–base abnormalities*, with calculation of the *anion gap* helping to determine the underlying pathophysiology.

Historical Notes

Progress in our understanding of blood gases has arguably been slow, with these landmarks in the nineteenth and twentieth centuries:

- 1837: Magnus, the first person to show the presence of both oxygen (O_2) and carbon dioxide (CO_2) using quantitative techniques, found more O_2 and less CO_2 in arterial blood compared with venous blood. He concluded that CO_2 must be added during the circulation of blood and is therefore related to O_2 consumption and heat production.
- 1850: Paul Bert established that oxygen 'pressure' and 'content' were related to each other.
- 1904: Bohr described the effect of PCO_2 on the oxyhaemaglobin-dissociation curve (Bohr effect).
- 1930s: Linus Pauling outlined the chemistry of oxygen carriage.
- 1928: Acid–base balance and carbon dioxide chemistry remained an enigma until the work of Henderson at Harvard who realised that 'when acids are added to blood, the hydrogen ions (H^+) react with bicarbonate (HCO_3^-)

generating CO_2 which is excreted by the lung almost eliminating it'.

- 1896: The first electromagnetic measurement of hydrogen ion concentration ($[H^+]$) by a platinum electrode.
- 1909: The unit of pH introduced (blame going to Sorrensen who was tired of writing seven zeros in a paper on enzyme activity).
- 1925: Practical platinum electrodes appeared.
- 1931: Thermostatically regulated electrodes introduced.

Clinical Blood Gas Analysis and Blood Gas Analysers

After initial volumetric measurements of released O_2 and CO_2, manometric methods were developed (Van Slyke technique 1924), followed by cumbersome pH measurements by equilibration with different CO_2 concentrations (Astrup 1956). A commercial system using small samples was then produced by Radiometer in time to aid the management of respiratory failure in polio victims.

A *PCO_2 electrode* (a glass pH electrode bathed in water separated from the CO_2 source by a rubber membrane permeable to CO_2) was conceived of by Richard Stow (1957).

The *PO_2 electrode* came from Clark by adapting polarography with platinum cathode and anode contained by cellophane to exclude protein, and measuring O_2 tension by oxidation–reduction reactions which produce measurable electric currents.

The three-electrode system is the current gold standard for respiratory monitoring in critical care, providing direct measurements of pH, PCO_2 and PO_2 and calculated values of HCO_3 and base excess. Direct measurements of carboxyhaemoglobin saturation and electrolyte concentrations are also available.

Arterial Blood Gas Sampling/Arterial Puncture

Direct access to arterial blood is relatively easy given the variety of vessels available (radial, ulnar, femoral), and the devices used. Arterial cannulation may be preferred to intermittent arterial puncture if regular blood pressure monitoring

and/or frequent ABG analysis is needed. The radial artery is the preferred site for both, given that the larger arteries have no collaterals and damage to the vessel walls may result in significant morbidity. The Allen test for the patency of the corresponding ulnar artery is often recommended but rarely carried out and Slogoff's 1983 paper, 'On the safety of Radial Artery Cannulation in *Anaesthesiology* 59:42–47', concludes: 'The available evidence does not support routine use of Allen's test prior to radial artery puncture'.

Syringes preloaded with dry heparin have made collection more consistent, with less potential for error through dilution of an inadequate sample volume (<3 mL) by residual liquid heparin in the barrel of the syringe (0.2 mL) (Figure 12.1). Preheparinised capillary tubes are perhaps the most convenient method of collecting blood for sampling and are widely used.

Physiology of Gas Exchange and Definitions

Respiration encompasses the:

- Delivery of O_2/removal of CO_2 via gas exchange in the lungs
- Circulation of gases
- Transfer of gas at a cellular level

Ventilation is the process of moving gas through the respiratory tract.

Gas partial pressures encountered are as follows:

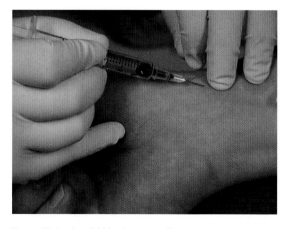

FIGURE 12.1. Arterial blood gas sampling.

- **In dry air** with a barometric pressure of 760 mmHg:

O_2 20.98%, i.e. $760 \times 0.21 = 160$ mmHg
  CO_2 0.04%
  N_2 78.06%
  Other gases 0.92%

Note the effect of different barometric pressures, for example, Salt Lake City 647 mmHg with PO_2 136 mmHg and the Dead Sea 775 mmHg with PO_2 163 mmHg

- **In moist air** (as in the respiratory tract) H_2O 47 mmHg makes the effective barometric pressure 760–47 = 713 mmHg. In **the alveolus** CO_2 at 40 mmHg displaces proportionate amounts of O_2 and N_2

Gas exchange is passive and dependent on small natural gradients across the alveolar membrane. A larger 'artificial' gradient exists for O_2 due to 'shunts' which allow deoxygenated, venous blood to bypass the lungs and dilute the oxygenated arterial blood. The bronchial and Thespian circulations are examples of anatomical shunts. The normal 'shunt fraction' is between 2% and 5% of the cardiac output and the resulting A-aO_2 gradient may be up to 15 mmHg.

Respiratory failure is defined as type 1 when there is hypoxaemia without carbon dioxide retention and type II when there is hypercapnia. Calculation of the gradient between the alveolar and arterial oxygen tensions (the A-a gradient) in type II respiratory failure will help to determine whether the patient has associated lung disease or just reduced respiratory effort.

Alveolar–Arterial Oxygen Gradient

$(A\text{-}a)PO_2 = PAO_2 - PaO_2$
$PAO_2 = PiO_2 - PACO_2/R$

Where R = respiratory quotient = volume of CO_2 produced/volume of O_2 consumed
R = 0.8 for a 'normal' diet and approaches 1.0 as proportion of carbohydrates consumed increases
$PiO_2 = (PB\text{-}PH_2O) \times FiO_2$
PiO_2 = partial pressure of inspired oxygen
PH_2O = water pressure
PB = barometric pressure
FiO_2 = fractional concentration of oxygen in inspired gas = 0.21 breathing air

Assuming PB = 101 kPa at sea level
  PH_2O = 6.2 kPa as inspired air is fully saturated by the time it reaches the carina
  Assume $PACO_2 = PaCO_2$ because of the ease of exchange of carbon dioxide
  Therefore:

$PAO_2 = (PB\text{-}PH_2O) \times FiO_2 - PaCO_2/R$
     $= (101-6.2) \times FiO_2 - PaCO_2/0.8$ (at sea level)
     $= 94.8 \times FiO_2 - 1.25 \times PaCO_2$

Breathing air, and with a $PaCO_2$ of 5.4 kPa

$PAO_2 = 94.8 \times 0.21 - (1.25 \times 5.48) = 12.25$ kPa

A raised $PaCO_2$ reflects reduced alveolar ventilation. Broadly speaking, this may be produced by a reduction in minute ventilation (central or peripheral pump failure), obstruction of airflow or a mismatch with perfusion giving a relative increase in dead space versus alveolar ventilation.

Disorders of the lung structure reduce the efficiency of oxygen transfer and widen the A-a gradient. The A-a gradient increases a little with age, but should be less than 2.6 kPa, so central respiratory depression should give a PaO_2 over 7.3 kPa in this situation. A PaO_2 below this signifies associated lung disease. Prolonged respiratory depression may lead to collapse of some areas of lung and an increase in the A-a gradient.

Oxygen Transport

Oxygen is largely transported bound to haemoglobin (Hb), with each gram of Hb capable of carrying 1.34 mL of O_2 (and hence 100 mL of blood with an average of 15 g of Hb, carries 20 mL of O_2 or 20 vol%). There are however subtle effects that bear on this capacity, including acid–base status whereby at a given PO_2, O_2 saturation is reduced by CO_2 (or acid) so that less O_2 is bound, and O_2 is usefully released, for example, in the capillaries where CO_2 is higher. This is graphically represented by a shift in the dissociation curve of Hb to the right—the *Bohr effect* (Figure 12.2).

Another useful alteration in the binding properties of O_2 and haemoglobin is the *Haldane effect*, where conformational changes in molecular subunits of Hb are induced by O_2 binding, making the histidine residues less ready to accept H^+. Deoxyhaemoglobin is thus a better H^+ acceptor than oxyhaemoglobin, allowing deoxyhaemoglobin to transport more CO_2 (i.e. H^+ and HCO_3^-).

Carbon Dioxide Transport

Carbon dioxide is transported by conversion to carbonic acid (H_2CO_3) and dissociation to H^+ and HCO_3^-. H^+ is buffered by Hb and HCO_3^- is taken up in plasma. As much as 12,000 nmol of CO_2 per day is thus transported to the lungs where H_2O and CO_2 are reconstituted and CO_2 expelled. These reactions are facilitated by carbonic anhydrase in red blood cells.

Acid–Base Status

At a cellular level the body, like all homeostatic systems, generally operates with a neutral pH of 6.8 and an alkaline blood pH of 7.4 at room temperature. Acids may accumulate to perturbate this equilibrium and are:

- Respiratory acid — CO_2. It is a volatile acid and can therefore be exhaled. Accumulation of CO_2 leads to a *respiratory acidosis.*
- Metabolic acids — all others. These may be neutralised, metabolised and/or excreted. Excess leads to a *metabolic acidosis* (in effect any reduction in pH *not* explained by a change in CO_2). A measure of this metabolic acid level, which is normally zero, is the lack of neutralising base or

put another way, a *negative base excess*, e.g. −10 (which is a metabolic acid excess of +10).

Additional definitions:
Normal $[H^+]$ — 36–44 nmol/L
Acidemia — $[H^+]$ above normal or pH < 7.4
Acidosis — A process that would cause acidemia if not compensated
Alkalemia — $[H^+]$ below normal or pH > 7.4
Alkalosis — A process that would cause alkalemia if not compensated

Normal Values

Traditionally, the measured values of pH and PCO_2 have been given a normal range based on traditional Gaussian statistics, i.e. 95% of the 'normal' population being covered by the mean ±2 standard deviations (SDs). It may be more reasonable however to consider the mean ±1SD (or 67% of the population) as being 'more' normal and is the one I have tended to use. In addition, if the pH and PCO_2 have 'normal' values bearing to opposite ends of the 'normal' range then I would at least consider this suggestive of a clinical perturbation in the system (Table 12.1).

Acid–Base Disturbances

There are two types of disorders, which may be uncompensated, partially compensated or fully compensated. Changes in pH that relate to changes

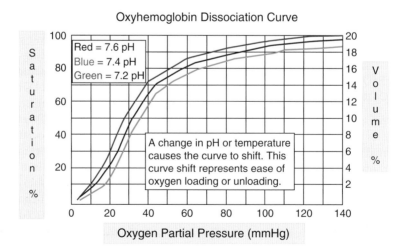

FIGURE 12.2. Oxyhaemoglobin dissociation curve.

TABLE 12.1. Normal values of arterial pH and $PaCO_2$

	Mean	1 SD	2 SD	Acceptable
pH	7.4	7.38–7.42	7.35–7.45	7.3–7.5
$PaCO_2$ (kPa)	5.3	5.0–5.6	4.7–6.0	4–6.7
HCO_3 mmols/L (calculated)	24	23.5–24.5	23–25	22–26

in PCO_2 are naturally termed respiratory disorders and conversely changes in pH brought about by changes in HCO_3^- are metabolic disorders. They are not uncommonly overlapping, e.g. respiratory acidosis as in COPD compensated through H^+ excretion and HCO_3^- reabsorption by the kidney, a metabolic alkalosis; or a metabolic acidosis as in renal failure compensated through hyperventilation, a respiratory alkalosis.

- *Respiratory acidosis* may be caused (commonly) by sedation or coma, respiratory muscle weakness/fatigue, airways obstruction or (rarely) lung restriction. Retention of CO_2 leads to production of HCO_3^- and H^+; however H^+ is buffered by proteins and Hb which limits the immediate fall in pH. In the acute phase HCO_3^- levels rise 1 mmol for every 1.3 kPa (10 mmHg) rise in PCO_2 with pH falling 0.05. Later H^+ excretion and further HCO_3^- reabsorption raises HCO_3^- by 4 for every increase in CO_2 of 1.3 kPa leading to compensation.
- *Respiratory alkalosis* or hyperventilation may be caused by anxiety, brain lesions, salicylates, acute asthma, pulmonary embolism or liver failure. Reduction in CO_2 drives the bicarbonate buffer system to produce carbonic acid through the release of H^+ from haemoglobin. The pH rise is limited by a 2 mmol fall in HCO_3^- for every reduction in PCO_2 of 1.3 kPa with pH rising 0.1. After some hours the kidney reduces H^+ excretion and HCO_3^- resorption (excretion increased) limiting the increase in pH. The HCO_3^- may be reduced by 5 mmol/1.3 kPa fall in CO_2 after 1–2 days.
- *Metabolic acidosis* may be caused by retention of excess acids of metabolic origin (diabetic, renal, lactic) or loss of alkali as in renal tubular lesions, or pancreatic fistula. Excess H^+ is buffered by Hb and by HCO_3^- leading to CO_2 production and hyperventilation. Hyperventilation may persist after resolution of the disorder because of the slow equilibration of CSF H^+.

- *Metabolic alkalosis* may be caused by loss of acid through vomiting, volume contraction associated with diuretic therapy or by ingestion of alkali (e.g. a high fruit diet). H^+ is released from Hb stores and CO_2 is retained by hypoventilation, though rarely causing the PCO_2 to rise to more than 7.3 kPa (55 mmHg) since oxygenation must be maintained

Base Excess

From the description of acid–base disorders in the section on 'Acid–Base Disturbances', it is obvious that CO_2 and HCO_3^- levels are intertwined and mixed acid–base disorders can be extremely difficult to dissect out if only pH, PCO_2 and (calculated) HCO_3^- values are available. In this situation the concept of base excess may help. This is the amount of acid that would be required to return the pH to 7.4 with the CO_2 at 5.3 kPa (40 mmHg). Normograms have been developed based on the experimental work of Siggard–Anderson, with positive base excess values indicating a metabolic alkalosis, and negative values a metabolic acidosis. Alternatively the pH expected for a given change in CO_2 above or below 5.3 kPa (40 mmHg) can be calculated (see Respiratory Acidosis and Respiratory Alkalosis), and simple compensation or another metabolic disturbance can therefore be recognised.

Anion Gap Concept

Organisms exist in a state of electrochemical neutrality with major and minor cations balanced by similar anions. The anion gap, $([Na^+ + K^+] - [HCO_3^- + Cl^-])$ is normally 10–20 mmol/L (or 8–16 mmol/L if K^+ is excluded), of which 11 mmol/L is typically due to albumin. A decreased calculated anion gap is usually caused by hypoalbuminaemia or severe haemodilution. Less commonly, it occurs as a result of an increase in minor cation concentrations such as in hypercalcaemia or hypermagnesaemia. Increased anion gap acidosis is caused by dehydration and by any process that increases the concentrations of lactate, ketones, renal acids or minor anions. It may also occur in patients being treated with organic salts, such as penicillin or salicylates, and in methanol or ethylene glycol toxicity. Rarely an increased anion gap may result from decreased minor cation concentrations such as calcium and magnesium.

Minor Anions and Cations

Cations	Anions
Potassium	Phosphates
Calcium	Sulphates
Magnesium	Organic anions such as proteins

Metabolic acidosis without an increased anion gap is typically associated with an increase in plasma chloride concentration (*hyperchloraemic acidosis*), and is usually caused by gastrointestinal loss or renal wasting of bicarbonate.

Oxygenation Disturbances

The range of normal values for PO$_2$ is less rigid than that for pH or PCO$_2$, and increasing age is associated with a decrease in PaO$_2$ values. A meta-analysis of studies done before the 1970s concluded that a reasonable prediction is provided by the equation PO$_2$ = 100 mmHg−1/3 age (years) (with PO$_2$ in mmHg = PO$_2$ in kPa × 7.5). Adult values for PO$_2$ and oxygen saturation (SaO$_2$) are given in Table 12.2.

The significance of these (arbitrary) values is evident on consideration of the sigmoid oxyhaemoglobin dissociation curve (Figure 12.2). Key points on the curve are listed in Table 12.3.

TABLE 12.2. Adult values for PO$_2$ and oxygen saturation

	PaO$_2$ (kPa)	SaO$_2$ (%)
Normal (range)	13 (≥10.7)	97 (95–100)
Hypoxaemia	<10.7	<95
Mild hypoxaemia	8–10.5	90–94
Moderate hypoxaemia	5.3–7.9	75–89
Severe hypoxaemia	<5.3	<75

TABLE 12.3. Key points on the oxyhaemoglobin dissociation curve

	Saturation (%)	PO$_2$ (kPa)
Normal	≅ 100	>12
Lower 'safe' level	90	8
Venous blood	75	6
Laboratory measurement (PO$_2$ at top of Everest)	50	4

When seeing a patient with a 'low' PO$_2$ it is reasonable to consider the mechanisms that might have brought this about, specifically:

- Low FiO$_2$ – will be evident (altitude)
- Hypoventilation and an increased PCO$_2$ (can be calculated)
- Diffusion barrier (unusual)
- Shunt
- Ventilation-perfusion imbalance

The only question to answer therefore is: 'Is this hypoventilation, i.e. is the PO$_2$ low only because the PCO$_2$ is high?', or put a different way: 'Is the A-a O$_2$ gradient normal?' (see Alveolar–Arterial Oxygen Gradient).

Clinical Approach to Blood Gas Interpretation

A structured approach to the interpretation of arterial blood gases helps ensure that nothing is missed. Two basic steps should be followed. Firstly, PaCO$_2$ and pH should be assessed. In essence this is the ventilatory state (respiratory acid–base balance) and will automatically lead to an assessment of the metabolic acid–base balance. Secondly, arterial oxygenation should be assessed. This includes evaluation of hypoxaemia as well as the arterial oxyhaemoglobin saturation along with the A-a gradient (Table 12.4).

TABLE 12.4. Systematic assessment of arterial blood gas measurements

Step 1a	Determine whether the PaCO$_2$ is low (<4.7 kPa) indicating alveolar hyperventilation, normal (4.7–6 kPa) or high (>6 kPa) as in ventilatory failure. Calculate the respiratory pH to determine if there is any metabolic compensation or additional disorder.
Step 1b	In the presence of a metabolic acidosis, calculate the anion gap to determine whether it has increased. No increase occurs with diarrhoea or urinary loss of bicarbonate.
Step 2a	Assess arterial oxygenation. Arterial hypoxaemia in adults is defined as PaO$_2$ < 10.7 kPa breathing room air, although it is not usually treated as clinically important unless below 8 kPa, when oxygen saturation will be 90% or less.
Step 2b	Calculate the A-a gradient to determine whether carbon dioxide retention is related to an intrapulmonary cause.

Alveolar hypoventilation (raised $PaCO_2$) with a normal pH probably represents a primary ventilatory change present long enough for renal mechanisms to compensate—as in chronic ventilatory failure. A similar picture can result from carbon dioxide retention from reduced ventilation compensating for a metabolic alkalosis, although such compensation is usually only partial. In acute respiratory failure the change in pH will be accounted for by the high carbon dioxide concentration.

Alternatively if the pH is appropriately raised for the reduction in the PCO_2 then acute alveolar hyperventilation is present. The renal system seldom compensates completely for an alkalosis, and the pH is often between 7.46 and 7.50 in chronic alveolar hyperventilation.

Alveolar hyperventilation (low $PaCO_2$) with a pH of 7.35–7.40 indicates a primary metabolic acidosis in which the respiratory system has normalised the pH. Although not impossible, it is very unusual for either the renal or the respiratory system to overcompensate. Alveolar hyperventilation in the presence of an arterial pH <7.35 suggests a severe metabolic acidosis or some limitation in the ability of the respiratory system to compensate.

A normal $PaCO_2$ accompanied by an arterial pH >7.45 represents a primary metabolic alkalosis to which the ventilatory system has not responded. In the presence of hypoxaemia, however, this might occur when patients with chronic carbon dioxide retention increase their usual level of ventilation. This may be seen when pulmonary emboli occur in chronic lung disease such as chronic obstructive pulmonary disease.

Controversies

Temperature Correction

When blood is cooled, CO_2 becomes more soluble reducing the PCO_2 by about 5% for every degree centigrade fall. With this the pH rises to 0.015/°C. Consequently with hypothermia, pH increases, PCO_2 falls and HCO_3^- is unchanged. This is important with regard to homeostasis, since the fractional dissociation of imidazole-histidine (α-imidazole) remains constant with changing pH if this is secondary to a change in temperature (α stat regulation).

pH/PCO_2 values are reported at 37°C and uncorrected for the patient's temperature (the α stat concept). pH/PCO_2 values can be corrected to the patient's (core) temperature (the pH stat concept). With few exceptions (e.g. deep hypothermic circulatory arrest) the appropriate clinical interpretation of ABGs is uncorrected.

Capillary Blood Gases

Arterial sampling is not risk free and may be painful. Whilst capillary sampling avoids potential arterial damage, values are altered by the non-arterial nature of the blood. This is related to normal arterio-venous differences: $PO_2 \sim 8\,kPa$ lower, (13→5), pH ~ 0.02 lower, $PCO_2 \sim 0.60\,kPa$ higher. The differences in pH and PCO_2 are acceptable for clinical use.

[H⁺] or pH?

pH is the negative $\log_{10}$ of H^+ concentration in nmol/L ([H^+] = 10^{-pH})

Although complex mathematically, these values can however be related by rule of thumb (Burden).

Conversion range pH 7.10–7.60, [H^+] 79–25 nmol/L

Treat the two decimal digits of pH as whole numbers, i.e. 7.10–7.60 = 10–60.

Subtract these from 83 to give [H^+] or 83 − [H^+] = pH 7.___

Pulse Oximetry—Artefacts? (Table 12.5)

The development of simple oximeters to measure oxygen saturation has been important in improving monitoring of oxygen therapy. The sigmoid saturation curve for haemogobin defines the relation between saturation and PaO_2. Oximeters work on the principle that desaturated haemoglobin and oxygenated haemoglobin absorb light of

TABLE 12.5. Problems with readings of pulse oximeters

Clinical situation	Result
Carboxyhaemoglobin	Falsely high saturation
Melanotic skin	Variable, reduced signal
Poor peripheral perfusion	Low signal, unreliable results
Severe pulmonary hypertension	Very low value due to pulsed venous signal

different wavelengths. The current devices use two wavelengths and measure the absorption in the pulsatile element of the blood flow, thus producing a measure of the oxygen saturation of arterial blood separate from the non-pulsatile venous blood. The probe is applied to the finger or earlobe. The delay in registration of central changes in saturation depends on the circulation time from the lungs to the monitoring site, with a finger probe registering a change approximately 30 s later than an ear probe. Oximeters tend to be less accurate with saturations below 75%, but for most clinical situations changes above this range are more important. Some clinical situations can affect the accuracy of measurement.

Further Reading

1. Henderson LJ. *Blood*. New Haven, CT: Yale University Press; 1928.
2. Williams AJ. Assessing and interpreting arterial blood gases and acid–base balance. *BMJ*. 1998;317:1213–1126.
3. Slogoff S, Keats AS, Arfund C. On the safety of radial artery cannulation. *Anaesthesiology*. 1983;59:42–47.
4. Siggaard Andreson O, Engel R, Jorgensen K, Astrup P. A micro method for determination of pH, carbon dioxide tension, base excess and standard bicarbonate in capillary blood. *Scand J Clin Lab Invest*. 1960;12:172–176.
5. Severinghouse JW, Astrup P, Murray JF. Blood gas analysis and critical care medicine. *Am J Respir Crit Care Med*. 1998;157 (4):5114–5122.

13
Inspired and Expired Gas Monitoring

Terry Fox

Abstract In this chapter the techniques used to monitor inspired/expired oxygen, carbon dioxide, nitric oxide and nitrogen dioxide in the critically ill are described. The importance of each parameter in the clinical setting is outlined. Derivation of resting energy expenditure (REE) from measurement of oxygen consumption and carbon dioxide production is also considered.

Introduction

Inspired oxygen concentration is routinely monitored in all critically ill patients, and in conjunction with the measurement of arterial oxygen saturation (SaO_2) and arterial oxygen tension (PaO_2) allows oxygen therapy to be optimised in individual cases. Expired carbon dioxide (CO_2) concentration, although not universally monitored, is being increasingly used to confirm successful endotracheal or inadvertent oesophageal intubation and to detect accidental disconnection from the ventilator. Metabolic rate can also be estimated from measurements of oxygen consumption and carbon dioxide production. In patients receiving inhaled nitric oxide for pulmonary hypertension or hypoxia due to adult respiratory distress syndrome (ARDS), it is mandatory to monitor both inhaled nitric oxide (NO) concentration and expired nitrogen dioxide (NO_2). Fortunately, our ability to monitor these gases has been greatly improved by advances in gas analyser technology, and these devices are now more precise, reliable and generally require less-frequent calibration than in the past.

Inspired Oxygen Gas Analysers

Although a number of different techniques may be used to monitor inspired oxygen concentration, the two most commonly used devices are the ambient temperature electrochemical sensor and the paramagnetic sensor. Users are encouraged to evaluate the merits of a particular sensor in relation to the context in which it is to be used.

Ambient Temperature Electrochemical Sensor

The sensor used most widely is the ambient temperature electrochemical sensor, which is often found in mechanical ventilators and portable oxygen analysers. Its main advantages are low cost and reliability. The sensor is typically a small, cylindrical, partially sealed device that contains two dissimilar electrodes immersed in an electrolyte solution, usually potassium hydroxide. As oxygen molecules diffuse through the semipermeable membrane installed on one side of the sensor, they are reduced at the cathode to form negatively charged hydroxyl ions. These then migrate to the anode where an oxidation reaction takes place. This process generates an electrical current proportional to the oxygen concentration of the gas sample. The current generated is both measured and conditioned with external electronics, and displayed on the screen of the oxygen analyser as percent oxygen or parts per million (ppm) concentration (Figure 13.1).

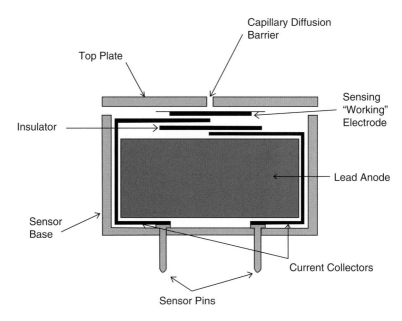

FIGURE 13.1. Schematic representation of an electrochemical oxygen sensor.

Paramagnetic Oxygen Sensor

The paramagnetic oxygen sensor is more commonly used in the industrial setting, since it has the ability to measure very low concentrations of oxygen. Although the device is expensive it is incorporated into some medical equipment, such as metabolic calorimeters, where sensitive and accurate oxygen analysis is required. As a highly paramagnetic gas, oxygen is readily attracted into magnetic fields. Indeed the degree to which oxygen becomes magnetised is several hundred times greater than most other gases such as nitrogen, helium and argon. In the sensor, a small glass dumb-bell is housed within a cylindrical casing. The dumb-bell contains an inert gas, such as nitrogen, and is suspended within a non-uniform magnetic field by a taught platinum wire. When a gas sample containing oxygen is passed through the sensor, oxygen molecules are attracted to the stronger of the two magnetic fields, causing the dumb-bell to rotate. An optical light source, photodiode and an amplifier are used to measure the degree of rotation, and an opposing current is applied to restore the glass dumb-bell to its normal position. The magnitude of the current required to keep the glass dumb-bell in its normal position is directly proportional to the partial pressure of oxygen in the gas sample. The partial pressure of oxygen can then be represented on an electronic screen as percent oxygen (Figure 13.2).

Datex Ohmeda Deltatrac™ Metabolic Calorimeter

The energy content of food can be determined by measuring the heat released during its combustion. This process of direct calorimetry utilises oxygen whilst producing carbon dioxide. Indirect calorimetry, a technique first reported by Benedict and Atwater in the early twentieth century, is the accepted method of measuring energy expenditure and substrate utilisation in humans, and requires the accurate measurement of oxygen consumption (VO_2) and carbon dioxide production (VCO_2). This information can be obtained using a metabolic calorimeter, such as the Datex Ohmeda Deltatrac™. The majority of indirect calorimeters feature mixing chambers and measurements can be performed in mechanically ventilated patients or in spontaneously breathing patients using a canopy, mouthpiece or mask. Expired gas from the patient is directed into the mixing chamber where baffles interrupt flow and prevent

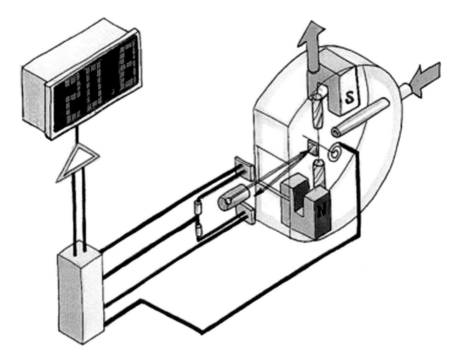

FIGURE 13.2. Schematic representation of a paramagnetic oxygen sensor.

streaming of gases and uneven gas concentration. At the end of the mixing chamber a vacuum pump withdraws a small sample of the mixed expired gas for measurement of oxygen and carbon dioxide concentrations (FEO_2 and $FECO_2$). Oxygen concentration is measured by a paramagnetic oxygen sensor and carbon dioxide using infrared absorption. The Deltatrac™ then applies the Weir equation to determine energy expenditure and displays this on a visual display unit (VDU) along with percent oxygen, VCO_2 (mL/min/m^2) and VO_2 (mL/min/m^2) (Figures 13.3 and 13.4).

Expired Carbon Dioxide Gas Analysers

Capnometry is the measurement and display of exhaled CO_2 concentration, usually as a percentage or partial pressure, whilst the graphical representation of this over time is known as capnography. A variety of techniques can be used to measure CO_2 in respiratory gases including mass spectroscopy, where expired gases are separated according to molecular weight, Raman spectroscopy, infrared spectroscopy and colorimetric devices. The latter

technique is the simplest, and uses pH sensitive indicators which change colour in response to different concentrations of CO_2. The colorimetric detector is placed between the endotracheal tube and ventilator. It remains purple in room air and turns yellow in the presence of CO_2. This reaction is reversible and therefore colour changes occur with each inspiration and expiration.

End tidal CO_2 (ETCO$_2$), the level of CO_2 at the very end of expiration, is the most commonly monitored measurement of expired CO_2. It is also the maximum concentration of expired CO_2 and is usually obtained using infrared spectroscopy. ETCO$_2$ can be monitored continuously in ventilated or non-ventilated patients using main-stream or side-stream devices, some of which are hand-held and particularly useful when transporting ventilated patients between hospital departments.

Infrared ETCO$_2$ Monitoring

Gases, such as CO_2, that contain molecules with at least two dissimilar atoms absorb infrared radiation. The wavelength maximally absorbed by CO_2 is 4.3 mm. An end-tidal CO_2 monitor consists of a

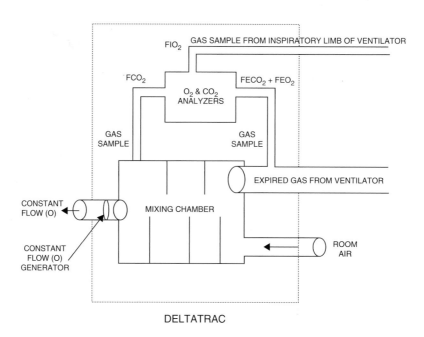

FIGURE 13.3. Schematic representation of the mixing chamber technique to measure inspired and expired gases.

THE WIER EQUATION

REE = [3.9(VO2) + 1.1(VCO2)] 1.44

REE = Resting energy expenditure
VO2 = Oxygen uptake (ml/min/m^2)
VCO2= Carbon dioxide output (ml/min/m^2)

3.9, 1.1 and 1.44 = constants

FIGURE 13.4. The Weir equation used to calculated resting energy expenditure (REE).

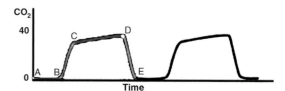

FIGURE 13.5. A typical waveform for expired CO_2. A to B: baseline CO_2. B to C: combination of dead space and alveolar gases. C to D: mostly alveolar gas. D: end of expiration and maximum expired or end-tidal CO_2 (ETCO$_2$). D to E: inspiration begins and CO_2 concentration rapidly falls to baseline.

light source emitting radiation at this wavelength and a photodetector to determine how much of the radiation is absorbed by the sample gas. According to the Beer–Lambert law, the amount of radiation absorbed is proportional to the number of CO_2 molecules present in the gas sample. This allows the concentration of CO_2 to be measured. A capnograph is obtained by measuring CO_2 concentration continuously throughout the respiratory cycle (Figure 13.5).

Mainstream ETCO$_2$

Mainstream ETCO$_2$ analysers use a sample chamber (glass cuvette) positioned between the patient's endotracheal tube and breathing circuit which allows inhaled/exhaled respiratory gases to pass through it. An infrared CO_2 sensor is then placed over the glass cuvette which allows for continuous monitoring of CO_2. There is no need for gas sampling as the glass cuvette is in line. The glass cuvette is heated above body temperature to ensure that no condensation forms which could interfere with the CO_2 analysis. CO_2 is displayed as a waveform with a numerical value on a visual display unit. Before use the ETCO$_2$ monitor must be calibrated with two known reference concentrations of CO_2.

FIGURE 13.6. Photograph of the INOvent nitric oxide delivery system connected to a mechanical ventilator.

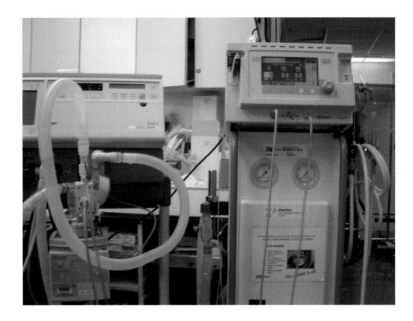

Sidestream ETCO$_2$

When using the side-stream technique, respiratory gases are drawn by a pump through a Teflon manometer line which runs from the endotracheal tube (or face mask if the patient is not mechanically ventilated) into a sampling module. Once inside the sampling chamber CO$_2$ concentration is analysed in the standard fashion using infrared spectroscopy. With this method respiratory gases must be sampled frequently in order to obtain a capnograph.

Inhaled Nitric Oxide

Nitric oxide (NO) is a colourless gas which is both diffusible and toxic. It is formed naturally within vascular endothelial cells from L-arginine and molecular oxygen in a reaction catalysed by NO synthase. NO then activates chemicals which lead to the relaxation of vascular smooth muscle. Inhaled NO selectively dilates pulmonary vessels in ventilated regions of the lung, thereby reducing V/Q mismatching and improving oxygenation. It also reduces pulmonary artery pressure and vascular resistance. Due to these properties it can be used to treat lung disorders, such as acute respira-

tory distress syndrome (ARDS) that are characterised by hypoxaemia and pulmonary hypertension. Inhaled NO is rapidly deactivated after diffusing into the blood stream by reacting with haemoglobin to form methaemoglobin and therefore has no effect on the systemic circulation.

Technological advances in the measurement of inhaled nitric oxide (NO) and expired nitrogen dioxide (NO$_2$) have rendered chemiluminescence obsolete, and both gases are now routinely measured using electrochemical cells. NO is inhaled via a ventilator circuit or face mask during the inspiratory phase of the respiratory cycle. When administered through a ventilator a continuous or intermittent flow of the gas is fed into the inspiratory limb of the ventilator circuit, and the flow rate is controlled so that the desired inspired concentration of NO is achieved. NO concentration levels are measured using a sampling line, placed close to the patient in the inspiratory limb of the circuit, and connected to a NO monitor which analyses NO and NO$_2$ in parts per million (ppm). Typically, NO concentrations of 5–40 ppm are used.

Although a number of different delivery systems are available the system manufactured by Inovent™, which encompasses NO, NO$_2$ and O$_2$ analysers, is the most common NO delivery system in use today (Figure 13.6).

Further Reading

1. http://.aoi- corp.com/additional_ information/oxygen analysers _ sensor _ types/
2. Walsh TS. Recent advances in gas exchange measurement in intensive care patients. *Br J Anaesth.* 2003;91: 120–131.
3. Branson RD, Johannigman JA. The measurement of energy expenditure. *Nutr Clin Pract.* 2004;19: 622–636.
4. St. John RE. End–tidal carbon dioxide monitoring. *Crit Care Nurse.* 2003;23:83–88.
5. http://www.nda.ox.ac.uk
6. Bhende MS. End-tidal carbon dioxide monitoring in paediatrics: concepts and technology. *J Postgrad Med.* 2001;47:153–156.
7. http://classes.kumc.edu.cahe/respcared/cybercas/nitricoxide/nother/html
8. http://www.euroanesthesia.org/education/rc_vienna/12rc7.HTM

14

Managing Secretions in the Ventilated Patient: The Role of Humidification, Suction, Physiotherapy, Mucolytics and Airway Adjuncts

George Ntoumenopoulos

Abstract Intubation and mechanical ventilation may impair secretion clearance, adversely affect respiratory mechanics and gas exchange, and lead to significant pulmonary complications. This chapter reviews the monitoring and impact of airway secretions in the intubated patient, and describes a number of techniques used to optimise secretion clearance including humidification, suction, physiotherapy, mucolytics and the use of airway adjuncts.

Airway Secretions and the Intubated Patient

Intubation and mechanical ventilation impair secretion clearance and can lead to lung collapse, consolidation and ventilator-associated pneumonia.[1,2] Normally, airway patency is maintained through mucociliary clearance and cough; however, during intubation and mechanical ventilation enhanced expiratory flow through two-phase gas–liquid transport becomes an essential means of airway clearance.[3,4] In addition to the existence of higher expiratory than inspiratory flows, dynamic airway compression also facilitates secretion clearance.[4]

Poor or absent cough as a result of sedation, paralysis and/or disease can impact on the ability to maintain adequate ventilation and gas exchange. For example, repositioning a heavily sedated patient with excessive airway secretions from supine to side-lying while ventilated in a pressure-controlled mode may result in significant reductions in tidal volume, arterial desaturation and hypercarbia. The effect of airway secretions on tidal volume, gas exchange and patient work of breathing may depend on the volume and location of the secretions in the patients' airway, extent of ventilation/perfusion (V/Q) mismatch caused by the secretions, pre-existing pulmonary disease (unilateral or bilateral lung pathology), the mode of mechanical ventilation (volume or pressure-controlled, including level of positive end-expiratory pressure [PEEP]), the patients' respiratory muscle strength and the position of the patient (e.g. head up, head down, side-lying). There is however no established link between airway secretions and patient morbidity/mortality.[5]

Monitoring of Airway Secretions

Even though monitoring of airway secretions with auscultation is unreliable, it can be useful to localise secretions and assist with therapy selection.[6] Clinical experience, patient habitus (e.g. morbid obesity), the auscultation tool, lung sound(s), point of auscultation, method of ventilation (spontaneously breathing vs. mechanically ventilated) and inspiratory/expiratory flow rates are all important factors affecting the accuracy of auscultation. Vibration response imaging (VRI) is a commercially developed acoustic lung imaging system that displays breath sound distribution, and may prove to be a useful clinical tool in identifying secretion retention.[7]

Airway secretions can also be detected by changes in respiratory mechanics at the bedside (i.e. increased airway resistance and reduced lung/thorax compliance). However, measurements of airway pressure and flow are often taken at the proximal end of the endotracheal tube (ETT), and are therefore affected by the mechanical properties of the ETT.[8] While the ability to locate secretions (e.g. ETT, major or peripheral airways) may be helpful in determining the intervention required (e.g. airway suction, physiotherapy, bronchoscopy or change of ETT), this has yet to be formally investigated. The presence of a sawtooth pattern in the expiratory flow waveform and coarse respiratory sounds over the trachea on expiration are good indicators of retained major airway secretions[9] (Table 14.1, Figure 14.1). ETT obstruction has a characteristic increase in early expiratory time constants.[8] Acoustic reflectometry is another means of detecting ETT obstruction, but is not easily applied in the clinical setting.[10,11]

Management of Airway Secretions

A recent paper by Branson provides a detailed review of the issues relevant to secretion management in the mechanically ventilated patient.[12] This chapter focuses on five key areas: humidification, suction, physiotherapy, mucolytics and airway adjuncts.

Humidification

Mechanical ventilation through an ETT bypasses the normal airway humidification systems, and

TABLE 14.1. Methods to detect airway secretions in intubated and ventilated patients

Detection of airway secretions
• Tracheal/chest wall auscultation (transmitted coarse sounds)
• Sawtooth expiratory waveform (real-time waveform analysis via ventilator)
• Chest palpation. If on low levels of respiratory support or poor inspiratory/expiratory flow rates, manually assist expiration with chest wall shaking/vibrations to increase expiratory flow rate. This will enhance detection of secretions visually via the waveform and on palpation of the chest wall
• ↑ Patient WOB, tachypnoea, diaphoresis, accessory muscle use, paradoxical respiration
• ↑ $PaCO_2$ (episodic or trends in data)
• Changes in ventilator parameters = ↓ TV, ↓ MV, ↓ Crs, ↑ PIP, ↑ Rrs (episodic or trends in data)
• Arterial desaturation (episodic or trends in data)

Abbreviations: WOB, work of breathing; PaCO2, partial pressure of carbon dioxide; TV, tidal volume; MV, minute volume; Crs, dynamic lung/thorax compliance; PIP, peak inspiratory pressure; Rrs, total airway resistance.

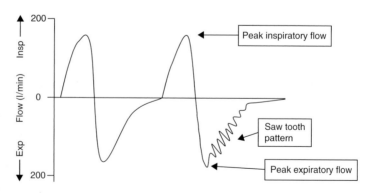

FIGURE 14.1. Flow/time curve with 'sawtooth pattern' and without airway secretions.

may cause structural and functional damage of the mucociliary escalator. Accumulation of inspissated secretions may also reduce ETT patency and cause obstruction.[13] The two most common forms of humidification used in the intubated patient are the heat and moisture exchanger (HME) and the heated humidifier.

HMEs are often advocated to reduce costs and the potential risk of ventilator-associated pneumonia.[14] However, the extended use of HMEs beyond 5 days of mechanical ventilation results in a 10% reduction in ETT patency and 30% increase in ETT airway resistance when compared with heated humidification.[13] HME devices also impair the mucus transport by cough.[15] In addition, unless adequate inspiratory assistance is provided, there can be an increase in the work of breathing in spontaneously breathing intubated patients.[16]

Airway Suction

Suction of an endotracheal or tracheostomy tube is recommended for secretion clearance and to maintain airway patency. The literature focuses on the safety of airway suction and minimising detrimental physiological effects.[17,18] Closed suction is often advocated as a means of minimising the detrimental effects of open suction (volume loss, hypoxaemia), but it may reduce the effectiveness of secretion removal.[17,19] Positive pressure ventilation (PEEP and/or pressure support) during closed suction may push secretions away from the suction catheter tip, and it may be necessary to revert to open suction or remove the PEEP/pressure support in order to improve secretion clearance.[17] Increased tenacity of secretions requires higher suction pressures and larger suction catheters, especially if closed suction is used.[17,20] Conventional volume-controlled ventilation may limit inspiratory gas flow during closed suction and improve secretion clearance; however, this may also result in greater lung de-recruitment.[21] Both the physical removal of secretions (suction pressure) and the 'pipe cleaner' effect of the suction catheter (hence larger catheters may be more useful) may be required to ensure patency of the ETT.[20]

Shortened suction catheters, designed to prevent contact with the carina, can minimise adverse physiological effects. One study, looking at a range of outcome measures, including duration of intubation, length of ICU-stay, ICU mortality and the incidence of pulmonary infections, found their performance to be equivalent to standard length catheters provided that the open method of suction is used.[22] However, it should be noted that in this study there were frequent protocol violations, with nurses opting to use standard length suction catheters when signs of secretion retention or arterial desaturation occurred.

Drugs that reduce consciousness and impair cough reflex/strength (sedation, narcotics, paralysing agents) may reduce the expiratory flow rate generated during normal airway care, and hence impair secretion clearance. Assessment of peak expiratory flow generated during secretion clearance procedures may assist clinicians to optimise therapy. The frequency of airway suctioning should be based on clinical need.[12]

Physiotherapy

A task force, with representatives from the European Intensive Care Medicine and European Respiratory Societies, recently reviewed the available literature on physiotherapy in the critically ill patient.[23] For secretion retention, the task force recommended use of head-down patient positioning, manual lung hyperinflation (MHI) or ventilator hyperinflation (VHI) and airway suctioning. A number of authors have also advocated the use of MHI/VHI, with and without chest wall vibrations, to improve secretion clearance, lung/thorax compliance and airway resistance.[12,23–28] Improved expiratory flow rate during lung hyperinflation and chest wall vibration probably explains the increased secretion clearance.[29,30] In relation to this, it is important to note that certain MHI circuits (e.g. Laerdal) when combined with PEEP above $10\,cmH_2O$ may retard expiratory flow to levels below that required for two-phase gas–liquid flow.[31] MHI is effective for secretion clearance up to the tenth generation of airways,[4] and head-down tilt may further enhance secretion clearance.[32–34]

The increased expiratory flow generated by disconnecting the patient from the ventilator for MHI or open suction (through elastic recoil) may also have beneficial effects on secretion clearance. Characterisation of the forces and flows generated during chest physiotherapy will help to optimise secretion clearance strategies[29] (Table 14.2).

TABLE 14.2.   Secretion management strategies in intubated/ventilated patients based on peak expiratory flow and/or cough response/abdominal contraction to airway suction (progressive increase in intervention based on patient response)

Abdominal contraction *present* on suction	Abdominal contraction *absent/poor* on suction
(Cough response should generate an expiratory flow bias)	(Cough response does not generate an expiratory flow bias)
1. Encourage voluntary deep breathing and cough to increase peak expiratory flow	1. Use chest wall vibrations/shaking followed by airway suctioning
2. If unable to cough voluntarily, use airway suction to stimulate a cough as required clinically (see Airway Suction)	2. Use two clinicians, one to deliver chest wall vibrations/shaking and the other to suction the airway during chest wall vibrations
3. Undertake passive/active limb and/or bed exercises, e.g. arm and/or leg exercises, with the aim of increasing minute ventilation and/or expiratory flow rates	3. Minimise the use of sedative/paralysing agents
4. Sit the patient over the edge of the bed to increase FRC and ability to cough voluntarily (ensure stable ETT/tracheostomy)	4. Treat in a supine, head-down position. Combine with suctioning before turning into side-lying to prevent aspiration of secretions into the dependent lung
	5. Combine MHI + head-down positioning/vibrations. Second person to assist cough/suction (may need open suction)
	6. MI-E ± assisted cough/suction
	7. Recommend PR-VC ventilation if episodic desaturation or tidal volume loss with patient repositioning due to secretion retention

Abbreviations: FRC, functional residual capacity; MI-E, mechanical in/exsufflation; PR-VC, pressure-regulated volume control.

Mobilisation of airway secretions, during chest wall vibrations in a paralysed animal model ventilated in a pressure-controlled mode, can cause deterioration in compliance and gas exchange.[34] Clinicians should be prepared for the potential adverse changes in ventilation, gas exchange and patient work of breathing during physiotherapy for secretion clearance and manage the scenario appropriately (e.g. prompt use of MHI may prevent airway occlusion).

Mucolytics

Mucus hypersecretion and plugging in the artificial or anatomical airways is common in the intubated patient.[2] Although mucolytics are frequently used clinically, there is scant evidence to support this practice,[35] and administration of some mucolytics may even worsen respiratory function. In particular, intra-tracheal instillation of Mesna (sodium salt of 2-mercaptoethane) can reduce arterial oxygen saturation and increase airway resistance and arterial carbon dioxide tension compared to saline lavage alone.[36] Other drugs, such as sublingually administered potassium dichromate, have been used to reduce secretion volume and may permit earlier extubation and shorten ICU length of stay in patients with a history of COPD and delayed weaning due to excessive airway secretions.[37]

Hendrik et al. retrospectively evaluated the effect of DNase, both instilled and nebulised, on the resolution of persistent atelectasis in a mixture of intubated and non-intubated paediatric patients and demonstrated significant improvement in 60% of patients.[38]

Endotracheal instillation of saline has been theorised to enhance secretion clearance through cough stimulation and some nebulous interactions between saline and mucus. Instillation of small volumes of saline (3 mL) can be used without compromising oxygenation or pulmonary mechanics.[36] However, larger volumes (5 mL) may cause short-term arterial desaturation.[39] Double-lumen suction devices (Irri-cath) that allow simultaneous saline infusion and aspiration have been shown to be more effective than conventional suctioning in clearing airway secretions without compromising oxygenation.[40] However, combining chest physiotherapy (MHI) with saline instillation may be a more effective means to clear secretions and maintain stable arterial saturation.[41]

There is very limited information on the use of *N*-acetylcysteine (NAC) as a mucolytic agent. It can be administered via a nebuliser or instilled directly into the airway, but may be associated with bronchospasm and worsening in gas exchange. Nebulised bronchodilators prior to NAC administration may ameliorate the bronchospasm.[42]

Physiotherapy Adjuncts

Peak cough expiratory flow (PCEF) is important for secretion clearance and falls with increasing age.[43] It is also impaired in patients with neuromuscular disease.[44] A PCEF of at least 160 L/min is required for effective clearance of airway secretions,[45] and values lower than this are associated with a greater risk of failed extubation in patients with neuromuscular disease.[46] Airway suction will trigger a cough and generate adequate expiratory flow under most circumstances, but may be less effective when respiratory muscle strength is impaired.

Mechanical in-exsufflation (MI-E) devices apply rapidly alternating positive and negative pressure to the airway via a mask, ETT or tracheostomy. The range of the pressure fluctuation is from –40 to +40 cmH$_2$O. This rapid shift in pressure generates a high expiratory flow rate simulating a cough. MI-E is often a more effective and less traumatic means of mobilising airway secretions in patients who cannot generate adequate peak cough expiratory flow (neuromuscular disease, sedated, paralysed). Most of the research relating to MI-E has been performed in non-intubated patients with severe neuromuscular diseases.[45,47] In a small study of six patients with amyotrophic lateral sclerosis, Sancho et al. reported improved arterial oxygen saturations following MI-E compared to conventional airway suction.[48]

Airway Adjuncts

Extubated patients who have difficulty clearing secretions may be helped by the insertion of a nasopharyngeal airway to facilitate airway suctioning. However, it should be noted that the benefits of this manoeuvre have not been investigated in a controlled fashion.[49] Portex® nasopharyngeal tubes are commonly used, with the average female needing a size 6 and male a size 7. Placement of the airway may be associated with increased cardiovascular stress, arrhythmias and local bleeding, and lubrication/warming of the tube may make insertion easier. In a minority of cases application of a topical vasoconstrictor and/or anaesthetic agent may be considered. The risk of intracranial placement in patients with a base of skull fracture is very low.[49]

Another technique, that may provide more effective airway access than a nasopharyngeal airway, is a mini-tracheostomy. This involves inserting a small-bore, cuffless tube through the crico-thyroid membrane into the trachea. It allows tracheal stimulation of cough and suction with small bore size

10 catheters, while preserving glottic function and avoiding conventional tracheostomy.[50] It cannot, however, prevent aspiration. Mini-tracheostomy may be usefully combined with non-invasive ventilation in patients with neuromuscular disease to reduce the need for formal intubation.[51]

References

1. Keller C, Brimacombe J. Bronchial mucus transport velocity in paralysed anesthetised patients: a comparison of the laryngeal mask airway and cuffed endotracheal tube. *Anesth Analg.* 1998;86:1280–1282.
2. Konrad F, Schreiber T, Brecht-Kraus D, Georgieff M. Mucociliary transport in ICU patients. *Chest.* 1994; 105:237–241.
3. Benjamin RG, Kim CS, Chapman GA, Sackner MA. Mechanical ventilation can move secretions by two-phase gas liquid transport. *Chest.* 1984; 86:284.
4. Kim CS, Sankaran S, Eldridge MA. Mucus transport by two-phase gas-liquid flow mechanism. *Am Rev Respir Dis.* 1984; 129:A313.
5. Hess D. The evidence for secretion clearance techniques. *Respir Care.* 2001;46:1276–1293.
6. Brooks D, Wilson L, Kelsey C. Accuracy and reliability of 'specialized' physical therapists in auscultating tape-recorded sounds. *Physiother Can.* 1993;45:21–24.
7. Dellinger R, Parrillo J, Kushnir A, Rossi M, Kushnir I. Dynamic visualisation of lung sounds with a vibration response device: a case series. *Respiration.* 2008;75:60–72.
8. Guttman J, Eberhard L, Haberthur C, et al. Detection of endotracheal tube obstruction by analysis of expiratory flow signal. *Intensive Care Med.* 1998;24:1163–1172.
9. Gugglielminotti J, Alzieu M, Maury E, Guidet B, Offenstadt G. Bedside detection of retained tracheobronchial secretions in patients receiving mechanical ventilation. *Chest.* 2000;118:1095–1099.
10. Boque M, Gualis B, Sandiumenge A, Rello J. Endotracheal tube intraluminal diameter narrowing after mechanical ventilation: use of acoustic reflectometry. *Intensive Care Med.* 2004;30:2204–2209.
11. Van Surrell C, Louis B, Lofaso F, et al. Acoustic method to estimate the longitudinal area profile of endotracheal tubes. *Am J Respir Care Med.* 1994;149:28–33.
12. Branson R. Secretion management in the mechanically ventilated patient. *Respir Care.* 2007;52:1328–1342.
13. Jaber S, Pigeot J, Fodil R, et al. Long term effects of different humidification systems on endotracheal tube patency. *Anesthesiol.* 2004;100:782–788.

14. Kola A, Eckerman T, Gastmeier P Efficacy of heat and moisture exchangers in preventing ventilator-associated pneumonia: meta-analysis of randomised controlled trials. *Intensive Care Med.* 2005;31:5–11.

15. Nakagawa N, Macchione M, Petrolino H, et al. Effects of heat and moisture exchanger and a heated humidification on respiratory mucus in patients undergoing mechanical ventilation. *Crit Care Med.* 2000;28:312–317.

16. Girault C, Breton L, Richard J-C, et al. Mechanical effects of airway humidification devices in difficult to wean patients. *Crit Care Med.* 2003;31:1306–1311.

17. Lindgren S, Almgren B, Hogman M, et al. Effectiveness and side-effects of closed and open suction: an experimental evaluation. *Intensive Care Med.* 2004;30:1630–1637.

18. Stiller K. Physiotherapy in intensive care. Towards and evidence-based practice. *Chest.* 2000;118:1801–1813.

19. Fernandez M, Piacentini E, Blanch L, Fernandez R. Changes in lung volume with three systems of endotracheal suction with and without pre-oxygenation in patients with mild-to-moderate lung failure. *Intensive Care Med.* 2004;30:2210–2215.

20. Morrow B, Futter M, Argent A. Endotracheal suction: from principles to practice. *Intensive Care Med.* 2004;30:1167–1174.

21. Masry A, Williams P, Chipman D, Kratohvil J, Kacmarek R. The impact of closed endotracheal suction systems on mechanical ventilator performance. *Respir Care.* 2005;50:345–353.

22. Leur JP, Zwaveling JH, Loef BG, Schans CP. Endotracheal suction versus minimally invasive airway suction in intubated patients: a prospective randomised controlled trial. *Intensive Care Med.* 2003;29:426–432.

23. Gosselink R, Bott J, Johnson M, et al. Physiotherapy for adult patients with critical illness: recommendations of the European Respiratory Society and European Society of Intensive Care Medicine Task Force on Physiotherapy for Critically Ill Patients. *Intensive Care Med.* 2008;34:1188–1199.

24. Berney S, Denehy L. A comparison of the effects of manual and ventilator hyperinflation on static lung compliance and sputum production in intubated and mechanically ventilated patients. *Physiother Res Int.* 2002;7:100–108.

25. Hodgson C, Denehy L, Ntoumenopoulos G, Santamaria J, Carroll S. An investigation of the early effects of manual hyperinflation in critically ill patients. *Anaesth Intensive Care.* 2000;28:492–496.

26. Choi J, Jones A. Effects of manual hyperinflation and suction in respiratory mechanics in mechanically ventilated patients with ventilator-associated pneumonia. *Aust J Physiother.* 2005;51:25–30.

27. Main E, Castel R, Newman D, Stocks J. Respiratory physiotherapy vs suction: the effects on respiratory function in ventilated infants and children. *Intensive Care Med.* 2004;30:1144–1151.

28. Maxwell L, Ellis E. Secretion clearance by manual hyperinflation: possible mechanisms. *Physiother Theory Pract.* 1998;14:189–197.

29. Gregson R, Stocks J, Petley G, et al. Simultaneous measurement of force and respiratory profiles during chest physiotherapy in ventilated children. *Physiol Meas.* 2007;28:1017–1028.

30. Maclean D, Drummond G, Macpherson C, Mclaren G, Prescott R. Maximum expiratory airflow during chest physiotherapy on ventilated patients before and after the application of an abdominal binder. *Intensive Care Med.* 1989;15:396–399.

31. Savian C, Chan P, Paratz J. The effect of positive end-expiratory pressure level on peak expiratory flow during manual hyperinflation. *Anesth Analg.* 2005;100:1112–1116.

32. Berney S, Denehy L, Pretto J. Head-down tilt and manual hyperinflation enhance sputum clearance in patients who are intubated and ventilated. *Aust J Physiother.* 2004;50:9–14.

33. Takahashi N, Murakami G, Ishikawa A, Sato T, Ito T. Anatomic evaluation of postural bronchial drainage of the lung with special reference to patients with tracheal intubation. *Chest.* 2004; 125:935–944.

34. Unoki T, Mizutani T, Toyooka H. Effects of expiratory rib cage compression combined with endotracheal suction on gas exchange in mechanically ventilated rabbits with induced atelectasis. *Respir Care.* 2004;49:896–901.

35. Rubin B. The pharmacologic approach to airway clearance: mucoactive agents. *Respir Care.* 2002;47:818–822.

36. Fernandez R, Sole J, Blanch L, Artigas A. The effect of short-term instillation of a mucolytic agent (Mesna) on airway resistance in mechanically ventilated patients. *Chest.* 1995;107:1101–110.

37. Frass M, Dielacher C, Linkesch M, et al. Influence of potassium dichromate on tracheal secretions in critically ill patients. *Chest.* 2005;127:936–941.

38. Hendrik T, Hoog M, Lequin M, Devos A, Merkus P. DNase and atelectasis in non-cystic fibrosis paediatric. *Crit Care.* 2005;9:351–356.

39. Ackerman MH and Mick DJ. Instillation of normal saline before suction on patients with pulmonary infections: a prospective randomised controlled trial. *Am J Crit Care.* 1998;7:261–266.

40. Isea J, Poyant D, O'Donnell C, Faling L, Karlinsky J, Celli B. Controlled trial of a continuous irrigation suction catheter vs conventional intermittent suction catheter in clearing bronchial secretions from ventilated patients. *Chest.* 1993;103:1227–1230.

41. Schreuder F, Jones U. The effect of saline instillation on sputum yield and oxygen saturation measurement in adult intubated patients: single subject design. *Physiotherapy*. 2004;90:108–109.

42. Jelic S, Cunningham J, Factor P. Airway hygiene in the intensive care unit. *Crit Care*. 2008;12:209 (doi:10.1186/cc6830).

43. Kim J, Davenport P, Sapienza C. Effect of expiratory muscle strength training on elderly cough function. *Arch Gerontol Geriatr*. 2008. Epub doi:10.1016/j. archger.2008.03.006.

44. Chiara T, Martin A, Davenport P, Bolser D. Expiratory muscle strength training in persons with multiple sclerosis having mild to moderate disability: effect on maximal expiratory pressure, pulmonary function and maximal voluntary cough. *Arch Phys Med Rehabil*. 2006;87:468–473.

45. Bach J, Ishikawa Y, Kim H. Prevention of pulmonary morbidity for patients with Duchene muscular dystrophy. *Chest*. 1997;112:1024–1028.

46. Bach J, Saporito L. Criteria for extubation and tracheostomy tube removal for patients with ventilatory failure: a different approach to weaning. *Chest*. 1996;110:1566–1571.

47. Chatwin M, Ross E, Hart N, Nickol A, Polkey M, Simonds A. Cough augmentation with mechanical insufflation/exsufflation in patients with neuromuscular weakness. *Eur Respir J*. 2003;21:502–508.

48. Sancho J, Servera E, Vergara P, Marin J. Mechanical insufflation-exsufflation vs. tracheal suction via tracheostomy tubes for patients with amyotrophic lateral sclerosis. *Am J Phys Med Rehabil*. 2003;82:750–753.

49. Roberts K, Whalley H, Bleetman A. The nasopharyngeal airway: dispelling myths and establishing the facts. *Emerg Med J*. 2005;22:394–396.

50. Balkan M, Ozdulger A, Tastepe I, Kaya S, Cetin G. Clinical experience with minitracheostomy. *Scand J Thorac Cardiovasc Surg*. 1996;30:93–96.

51. Vianello A, Bevilacqua M, Arcaro G, et al. Non-invasive ventilatory approach to treatment of acute respiratory failure in neuromuscular disorders. A comparison with endotracheal intubation. *Intensive Care Med*. 2000;26:384–390.

15
Drugs Acting on the Respiratory System

Gavin Whelan and Catherine McKenzie

Abstract This chapter describes a number of pharmacological agents used to treat respiratory disease in the critically ill. It includes respiratory stimulants, bronchodilators, corticosteroids, magnesium, pulmonary vasodilators and mucolytic agents. Where possible, evidence to support practice is included, although in some cases (e.g. mucolytic therapy) little evidence is available. Clinical applications are also described where relevant.

Respiratory Stimulants

Respiratory stimulants have limited use in the treatment of ventilatory failure, and Doxapram is the only example that remains in clinical use due to the increased incidence of seizures associated with earlier compounds.

Doxapram

Evidence

A Cochrane review published in 2002 concluded that doxapram had a marginal benefit over placebo in preventing blood gas deterioration, but that evidence comparing doxapram with non-invasive ventilation was conflicting.[1] An early trial suggested that it might be superior to non-invasive ventilation,[2] whilst a later, larger trial observed equal efficacy in terms of blood gas changes, treatment failures and mortality.[3]

Mode of Action

Doxapram increases minute volume by increasing respiratory rate and tidal volume, thereby decreasing $PaCO_2$ and increasing PaO_2. Although its precise mechanism of action is unknown, it is thought to act mainly through stimulation of peripheral chemoreceptors especially in the carotid body.[4]

Dosage Range

The recommended dosage range is 1.0–1.5 mg/kg administered as a slow bolus, repeated at hourly intervals if required.[5]

It may also be given as a continuous infusion at 1–4 mg/min, adjusted according to clinical response and blood gas measurements, although this route is unlicensed.[6]

Adverse Drug Reactions

Stimulation of the central, peripheral and autonomic nervous systems can occur even within the normal therapeutic range leading to muscle fasciculation, spasm, generalised seizures, hypertension and dysrhythmias.[4,5]

Pharmaceutical Problems

A combination of increased arousal and respiratory drive may enhance patient awareness of the bronchospasm and result in increased coughing.

Bronchodilators

Bronchodilator therapy is the mainstay of treatment in obstructive lung disease. The three classes of bronchodilators are β_2-adrenoreceptor agonists, anticholinergic agents and methylxanthines.

β_2-Adrenoreceptor Agonists

Evidence

Current national guidelines for asthma[7] and chronic obstructive pulmonary disease (COPD)[8] recommend the use of β_2-agonists as first-line agents for the treatment of acute exacerbations. In the treatment of acute severe asthma nebulised β_2-agonists are as efficacious, and in most cases preferable, to the intravenous route.[9] Continuous nebulisation should be reserved for cases of severe airflow obstruction or failure to respond to initial therapy.[10] Parenteral β_2-agonists in addition to a nebulised drug may have a role in the treatment of ventilated patients or those who have failed to respond to nebulised therapy alone. In the treatment of acute exacerbations of COPD, nebulised β_2-agonists may be used alone for moderate exacerbations, but in more severe cases should be combined with an anticholinergic bronchodilator.[11]

Mode of Action

The main effect of β_2-agonists is achieved through a direct action on the β_2-adrenoreceptors located in bronchial smooth muscle causing bronchodilation. A secondary action is inhibition of mediator release from mast cells, and they may also inhibit vagal tone and increase mucus clearance via an action on cilia.[4]

Dosage Range

The dosage ranges for β_2-adrenoreceptor agonists vary greatly and the reader is advised to consult the individual product literature for the most accurate information.

Adverse Drug Reactions

Adverse drug reactions do occur, usually in association with nebulised, oral or parenteral therapy, and are particularly frequent in critically ill patients. Tachycardia and palpitations, due to their

action on the β receptors located in cardiac tissue, are the main dose-limiting side effects. At the higher end of the dosage range, β_2-agonists may also cause hypokalaemia and worsening of angina. Other adverse effects associated with their use include fine tremor and peripheral vasodilation.[4]

Anticholinergics

Evidence

The National Institute for Clinical Excellence (NICE) recommends the use of anticholinergics in conjunction with β_2-agonists in patients with severe exacerbations of COPD, and in those who have responded poorly to β_2-agonists alone.[8]

In acute severe asthma the combination of an anticholinergic agent and β_2-agonist has been shown to produce greater bronchodilation than a β_2-agonist alone, leading to faster recovery and shorter length of stay.[11] For milder exacerbations, or for those patients who have already been stabilised, anticholinergic treatment is not necessary.

Mode of Action

Although their precise mechanism of action is unknown, it is most probably through competitive inhibition of cholinergic receptors located in bronchial smooth muscle. This antagonises the effects of acetylcholine, thereby blocking the bronchoconstricting action of vagal impulses, producing dilation of both large and small airways. Long-term use of anticholinergics has been associated with decreased sputum volume; however, anticholinergics have little or no effect on cilia motility, sputum viscosity or the rate of mucociliary clearance.[4]

Dose Range

Nebulised ipratropium 500 µg every 4–6 h

Adverse Drug Reactions

Adverse reactions to ipratropium are rarely seen in practice, as it is poorly absorbed from the lungs into the systemic circulation and does not cross the blood/brain barrier. The most common unwanted effects are dry mouth, sore throat and altered taste after nebulisation. Ocular side effects may occur if ipratropium is administered via a facemask instead of a mouthpiece allowing leakage of ipratropium into the eyes.[4]

Methylxanthines

Evidence

In the treatment of acute exacerbations of COPD, NICE recommends the addition of intravenous aminophylline for all patients who have failed to respond to bronchodilator therapy, although it acknowledges that there is little evidence for its use or effectiveness in these situations.[8]

For acute severe asthma little improvement is gained by adding aminophylline to optimised bronchodilator and steroid therapy. However, a small number of patients with life-threatening asthma who have failed to respond to other therapies may benefit from its addition. These patients are extremely rare, and were difficult to identify in a meta-analysis of 739 patients.[12]

Mode of Action

The mode of action of methylxanthines is uncertain, but is thought to include:

- An anti-inflammatory effect, probably achieved through one or more molecular mechanisms but not involving phosphodiesterase inhibition
- Immunomodulatory effects including suppression of neutrophils, eosinophils, eosinophil cationic protein and cytokine production. However, these effects are usually longer term, and are unlikely to play a major role in the acute phase
- Respiratory stimulation resulting in decreased resting end-tidal CO_2 and greater ventilatory and inspiratory effort in response to CO_2
- Bronchodilation through a wide variety of mechanisms[4]

Dosage Range

Aminophylline is a combination product of theophylline (85%) and ethylenediamine (15%). Aminophylline is the only intravenous formulation of theophylline. A loading dose of 5 mg/kg is given IV over 20 min, unless the patient is already receiving oral maintenance theophylline. This is followed by an infusion of 500–700 μg/kg/h.[4]

Adverse Drug Reactions

Adverse events occur more frequently and are more severe when therapeutic levels are exceeded. Common adverse events are anorexia, tremor, tachycardia and in more severe cases arrhythmia, hyperkalaemia and seizures.[13]

Pharmaceutical Problems

Aminophylline has a narrow therapeutic range, and regular monitoring of levels is recommended. The usual target plasma range is 10–20 mg/L, although in patients with hypoalbuminaemia salivary free theophylline level (range 5–10 mg/L) is more accurate. All patients receiving aminophylline infusions should have a level taken daily. Caution must be used in patients with heart failure or cirrhosis as the half-life of theophylline is increased. The half-life is reduced in smokers.

Corticosteroids

Evidence

Although corticosteroids are routinely used in the management of acute severe asthma, the evidence supporting high or low doses has been conflicting. A Cochrane review has helped to clarify this issue, by examining the use of low-, medium- and high-dose regimens. It concluded that there were similar outcomes in all treatment groups, and therefore the lowest dose regimens should be prescribed. However, the trials included in the review excluded patients requiring ventilatory support, and therefore the conclusions may not be applicable in the critically ill.[14]

In the treatment of COPD corticosteroids have favourable effects on FEV_1,[15] and lead to significant improvements in arterial PaO_2.[16] Patients receiving corticosteroids also have a shorter length of hospital stay,[17] although no effect on mortality has been observed.[15]

Mode of Action

The pharmacology of corticosteroids is complex. After entering a cell, they bind to specific receptors in the cell nucleus, causing activation and exposure of DNA-binding domains. The steroid–receptor complex then binds to the target DNA and either induces or inhibits transcription of the target gene. There are believed to be between 10 and 100 steroid responsive genes in each cell, and this explains the wide range of effects seen with steroid use. Gluco-corticoids are attributed with three main effects:

- General metabolic and systemic effects including increased protein metabolism and gluconeogen-esis together with decreased protein synthesis and utilisation of glucose
- Negative feedback on the anterior pituitary and hypothalamus decreasing endogenous corticos-teroid production
- Anti-inflammatory and immunosuppressive effects including both the early and late mani-festations of inflammation[18]

Dosage Range

For the treatment of exacerbations of COPD national guidelines recommend the use of 30 mg prednisolone daily for 7–14 days. No benefit is obtained from continuing treatment beyond 14 days.[8] For acute exacerbations of asthma 40–50 mg prednisolone daily or 100 mg parenteral hydrocortisone every 6 h is recommended for 5 days or until recovery,[7] and it is not uncommon to use up to 200 mg hydrocor-tisone IV every 6 h in the ventilated patient.

Adverse Drug Reactions

Corticosteroids have an extensive range of side effects. The most relevant in the critical care setting are adrenal suppression after long-term administration (this is important when consider-ing the patient's response to stress such as major surgery), gastrointestinal bleeding, diabetes, salt and water retention and proximal myopathy. Other common side effects include osteoporosis after long-term administration, disturbances in mental state and increased susceptibility to infections.[19]

Magnesium

Evidence

A Cochrane review, looking at the use of systemic magnesium in the emergency room for treatment of acute asthma, failed to show a significant benefit in terms of admission rates or pulmonary function for pooled results. Analysis of those patients with severe asthma did demonstrate benefit, although the clinical significance of this was difficult to determine.[20]

Current national guidelines recommend the use of a single dose of magnesium for all patients with acute severe asthma who have responded poorly to initial bronchodilator therapy or have life-threatening asthma.[7]

Several studies have also examined the use of inhaled magnesium in the treatment of acute asthma. A Cochrane review of the trials concluded that the use of nebulised magnesium in addition to nebulised β_2-agonists did appear to show benefit in patients with severe asthma, but more robust research is needed to provide a definitive answer.[21]

Mechanism of Action

The exact mechanism of action of magnesium in the treatment of asthma is unknown. It is thought to decrease the uptake of calcium by bronchial smooth muscle, leading to bronchodilation, and is also known to inhibit mast cell degranulation.[22]

Dosage Range

A single dose of 1.2–2 g of magnesium should be infused over a period of 20 min.[7]

Pulmonary Vasodilators

Indications for Use

The two main indications for pulmonary vasodila-tors in the critically ill are acute respiratory distress syndrome (ARDS) and pulmonary arterial hyper-tension. This section describes the use of inhaled nitric oxide (iNO), in ARDS specifically, and a number of other inhaled and systemic pulmonary vasodilators in pulmonary hypertension.

Inhaled Nitric Oxide (Medical Gas)

Inhaled nitric oxide (iNO) is used as a pulmonary vasodilator in critically ill patients with severe ARDS and/or pulmonary hypertension.

Mode of Action

NO is a potent endogenous, endothelium-derived vasodilator that directly relaxes vascular smooth muscle through stimulation of soluble guanylate cyclase and increased production of intracellular cyclic guanosine monophosphate (cGMP). In ARDS, iNO selectively dilates blood vessels supplying ventilated regions of the lung, thus reducing ventilation/perfusion (V/Q) mismatch and improving oxygenation.

Delivery of Nitric Oxide

The following should be in place to ensure safe delivery of iNO:

1. A continuous or synchronised inspiratory injection device
2. A calibrated flow metre
3. iNO/N_2 delivered into the ventilator circuit as close to the patient as possible

Dosing of iNO

The dose required to produce a reduction in pulmonary artery pressure is higher than that needed to improve PaO_2 in ARDS. In ARDS the dose used is usually between 5 and 20 parts per million (ppm), whilst 20–40 ppm may be required to treat pulmonary hypertension.

When iNO is started for refractory hypoxia in ARDS, a dose response test should be performed, to identify the minimum dose required to achieve a 20% improvement in PaO_2. An example of this can be seen in Table 15.1. About a third of patients will not gain any significant benefit from iNO, and it should be discontinued without undue delay in these cases.

TABLE 15.1. Example of a dose response test for the use of inhaled nitric oxide (iNO) in acute respiratory distress syndrome (ARDS)

Time (min)	Dose (ppm)	Response
60	5	Use the minimum dose required
60	10	to produce a 20% improvement
60	20	in PaO_2

The response to NO at each dose should be considered cumulative. The desired response is an overall increase of 20% from lowest to highest dose.

Nitric Oxide Withdrawal

There are reports of severe rebound hypoxemia and pulmonary hypertension following withdrawal of therapy. Slow withdrawal of treatment in a decremental fashion is advisable, e.g. dose is halved for 12 h then stopped. Use of systemic therapies (bosentan or sildenafil) may be helpful in severe cases.[23]

Severe ARDS

iNO improves oxygenation and reduces pulmonary artery pressure in the majority of patients with ARDS.[24] Evidence that iNO improves outcome in terms of mortality is scant, despite a number of major randomised placebo-controlled studies.[25,26] In our institution iNO is reserved for those ARDS patients with a P/F ratio (PaO2: FiO2) of <12 KPa in whom a number of other strategies may already have been tried:

- Recruitment manoeuvre
- Prone positioning
- High frequency oscillation

Pulmonary Artery Hypertension

iNO has been used in pulmonary artery hypertension to decrease pulmonary vascular resistance and therefore right heart afterload. Although there have been favourable case reports, there have been no prospective controlled studies to date.[27–29]

Monitoring During iNO Therapy

Methaemoglobin levels should be monitored at 0, 1 and 6 h and then daily. NO and NO_2 must be continuously monitored at the ventilator Y-piece, using electrochemical monitors with appropriate calibration.

Contraindications to Therapy

Absolute: methaemoglobinaemia
Relative: bleeding diatheses, intracranial haemorrhage

Prostaglandins

Prostaglandins are potent pulmonary vasodilators and inhibitors of platelet aggregation. They are also known to have cytoprotective and anti-proliferative properties. The two agents currently available for clinical use in the United Kingdom are Prostacyclin (PGI_2) and iloprost. In the following sections their role in managing pulmonary hypertension in the critically ill is described.

Intravenous Prostacyclin (PGI₂)

PGI_2 is synthesised from arachidonic acid in the vascular endothelium, and induces vascular smooth muscle relaxation through stimulation of cyclic AMP production.

Intravenous PGI_2 can be used to treat pulmonary hypertension in doses ranging from 2 to 10 ng/kg/min, depending upon patient response and tolerance. Problems with increased right to left lung shunting (due to reduced hypoxic vasoconstriction), and systemic vasodilation may limit its usefulness in the critically ill. For chronic administration a long-term tunnelled catheter is required.

Inhaled PGI₂

There is evidence that inhaled PGI_2 is of benefit in the treatment of pulmonary hypertension, in terms of reducing mean pulmonary arterial pressure and improving oxygenation.[30] The inhaled route has several advantages, most importantly the vast reduction in systemic adverse effects and immediate delivery to its site of action. However, PGI_2 has a very short half-life of approximately 1–2 min, which means that it must be administered by continuous nebulisation. A constant rate of 8 mL/h of a 20,000 ng/mL solution has been quoted.[30] Continuous nebulisation can be very difficult to achieve in the unstable patient. Furthermore, its alkaline pH can result in local irritation and discomfort for the patient. The more stable analogue iloprost is now preferred in clinical practice

Inhaled Iloprost

Iloprost is a stable prostacyclin analogue with a $t_{1/2}$ of 20–30 min, which has been shown to be beneficial when inhaled in patients with pulmonary hypertension.[31,32] Its major advantage in critical illness is its longer half-life, hence intermittent nebulisation can be delivered via the ventilator. Furthermore, it has a lower pH than PGI_2 making it significantly less irritant by inhalation. Published studies have used doses of 2.5–10 mcg every 2–4 h.[4]

In clinical practice at Guy's and St. Thomas' NHS Foundation Trust, we have used doses as high as 50 mcg every 2–4h, with good clinical effect in terms of improved oxygenation and reduction in pulmonary artery pressure.

Enteral Therapies

Not surprisingly, there is little evidence for enteral therapies in the critically ill. There are however a number of studies demonstrating a benefit from enteral therapies, such as bosentan and/or sildenafil, in ambulant patients with pulmonary hypertension.[33,34]

Bosentan

Bosentan is a dual endothelin receptor antagonist. It blocks both Endothelium A and Endothelium B receptors. It is thus anti-proliferative and may be most useful in primary pulmonary hypertension. The starting dose is usually 62.5 mg twice daily, and is titrated up to 125 mg twice daily.

Sildenafil

Sildenafil is a phosphodiesterase 5 (PDE5) inhibitor that decreases guanyl mono-phosphate (cGMP) breakdown, thus enhancing the effect of endogenous nitric oxide. The starting dose is normally 50 mg/day, and is titrated up to 150 mg/day.

Mucolytic Agents

Mucolytic agents are used commonly in the critically ill patient, typically for mucous plugging in patients with very viscous secretions. There is a paucity of evidence for any of the agents currently used in clinical practice.

N-Acetylcysteine (NAC)

Mucus consists of mucoproteins held together by disulphide bonds. NAC breaks these double bonds and reduces its viscosity. Use of 10% solution nebulised 6 hourly may be helpful in asthmatics, but there are no controlled studies demonstrating benefit in this patient group.[35,36] NAC is a reducing agent and is destroyed by high oxygen concentrations, it is therefore ineffective in higher levels of inspired oxygen (>50%, FiO_2 0.5).[37]

The following solution is prepared for *N*-acetyl-cysteine nebulisation at Guy's and St. Thomas' NHS Foundation Trust:

- *N*-acetylcysteine 20% (2,000 mg in 10 mL injection) 4 mL
- Salbutamol 5 mg nebule 1 mL
- Sodium chloride 0.9% 3 mL

Nebulise 4 mL of this solution and discard the remainder.

Sodium Chloride

A number of strengths have been used in the critically ill from isotonic 0.9% sodium chloride to concentrations as high as 5%. There is little evidence for the use of any strength in the ventilated patient.

References

1. Greenstone M, Lasserson TJ. Doxapram for ventilatory failure due to exacerbations of chronic obstructive pulmonary disease. Cochrane Database of Systematic Reviews. 2002;Issue 2,Art. No.: CD000223. DOI: 0.1002/14651858.CD000223.
2. Angus RM, Ahmed AEA, Fenwick LJ, Peacock AJ. Comparison of the acute affects on gas exchange of nasal ventilation and doxapram in exacerbations of chronic obstructive pulmonary disease. *Thorax.* 1996;51(10):1048–1050.
3. Newman WJ, Banham SJ, Barr J, et al. A Randomised trial comparing non-invasive ventilation with the respiratory stimulant, doxapram, in the treatment of acute hypercapnic respiratory failure complicating exacerbations of chronic obstructive pulmonary disease. Unpublished data 2001.
4. *DRUGDEX® System* [database on CD-ROM]. Version 5.1. Greenwood Village, Colo: Thomson Reuters (Healthcare) Inc.
5. Summary of Product Characteristics Dopram® Injection. Anpharm Ltd. March 2001.
6. Kaufman L, Taberner PV. *Pharmacology in the Practice of Anaesthesia.* London: Edward Arnold; 1996.
7. British Thoracic Society, SIGN. British Guideline on the Management of Asthma. *Thorax.* 2008;63 (Suppl IV)
8. Chronic Obstructive Pulmonary Disease: National Institute of Clinical Excellence. *Thorax.* 2004;59 (Suppl):1–232
9. Travers A, Jones AP, Kelly K, Barker SJ, Camargo CA Jr., Rowe BH. Intravenous beta2-agonists for acute asthma in the emergency department. Cochrane Database of Systematic Reviews. 2001;Issue 2,Art. No.: CD002988. DOI: 10.1002/14651858.CD002988.
10. Innes NJ, Stocking, JA, Daynes TJ, Harrison BDW. Randomised pragmatic comparison of UK and US treatment of acute asthma presenting to hospital. *Thorax.* 2002;57(12):1040–1044.
11. Moayyedi P, Congleton J, Page RL, Pearson SB, Muers MF. Comparison of nebulised salbutamol and ipratropium bromide with salbutamol alone in the treatment of chronic obstructive pulmonary disease. *Thorax.* 1995;50:834–837.
12. Lanes SF, Garrett JE, Wentworth CE III, Fitzgerald MJ, Karpel JP. The effect of adding ipratropium bromide to salbutamol in the treatment of acute severe asthma: a pooled analysis of three trials. *Chest.* 1998;114: 365–372.
13. Parameswaran K, Belda J, Rowe BH. Addition of intravenous aminophylline to beta2-agonists in adults with acute asthma. Cochrane Database of Systematic Reviews. 2000;Issue 4,Art. No.: CD002742. DOI: 10.1002/14651858.CD002742.
14. Manser R, Reid D, Abramson M. Corticosteroids for acute severe asthma in hospitalised patients. Cochrane Database of Systematic Reviews. 2000; Issue 3,Art. No.: CD001740. DOI: 10.1002/14651858. CD001740.
15. Wood-Baker RR, Gibson PG, Hannay M, Walters EH, Walters JAE. Systemic corticosteroids for acute exacerbations of chronic obstructive pulmonary disease. Cochrane Database of Systematic Reviews. 2004; Issue 4,Art. No.: CD001288. DOI: 10.1002/14651858. CD001288.pub2.
16. Maltais F, Ostinelli J, Bourbeau J, et al. Comparison of nebulized budesonide and oral prednisolone with placebo in the treatment of acute exacerbations of chronic obstructive pulmonary disease: a randomized controlled trial. *Am J Respir Crit Care Med.* 2002;165: 698–703.
17. Niewoehner DE, Erbland ML, Deupree RH, et al. Effect of systemic glucocorticoids on exacerbations of chronic obstructive pulmonary disease. *NEJM.* 1999;340: 1941–1947.
18. Rang HP, Dale MM, Ritter JM, Moore P. In Pharmacology. 5th ed. Edinburgh: Churchill Livingstone; 2003.
19. British National Formulary 55th Edition. London: BMJ; March 2008.
20. Rowe BH, Bretzlaff JA, Bourdon C, Bota GW, Camargo CA Jr. Magnesium sulfate for treating exacerbations of acute asthma in the emergency department. Cochrane Database of Systematic Reviews. 1999; Issue 4,Art. No.: CD001490. DOI: 10.1002/14651858.CD001490.
21. Blitz M, Blitz S, Beasely R, et al. Inhaled magnesium sulfate in the treatment of acute asthma. Cochrane Database of Systematic Reviews. 2003;Issue 3,Art. No.: CD003898. DOI: 10.1002/14651858.CD003898.pub4.

22. Skobcloff EM. An ion for the lungs. *Acad Emerg Med.* 1996;3:1082–1085.

23. Behrends M, Beiderlinden M, Peters J. Combination of sildenafil and bosentan for nitric oxide withdrawal. *Eur J Anaesth.* 2005;22:154–163.

24. Cuthbertson BH, Dellinger P, Dyar OJ, et al. UK guidelines for the use of inhaled nitric oxide therapy in the adult ICUs. *Int. Care Med.* 1997;23:1212–1218.

25. Schwebel C, Beuret P, Pedrix JP, et al. (1997) Early nitric oxide inhalation in acute lung injury: results of a double blind randomised study. *Int Care Med.* 1997;23(1):5.

26. Lundin S, Mang H, Smithis M, Stenquist O, Frostel C. For the European Study Group of Inhaled Nitric Oxide. Inhalation of inhaled nitric oxide in acute lung injury: preliminary results of a European multicentered study. *Int Care Med.* 1997;23(1):6.

27. Rich GF, Murphy GD, Roos CM, Johns RA. Inhaled nitric oxide; selective pulmonary vasodilatation in cardiac surgery patients. *Anesthesiology.* 1993;78: 1028–1035.

28. Girard C, Lehot JJ, Pannatier J-C, Filley S, Ffrench P, Estanove S. Inhaled nitric oxide after mitral valve replacement in patients with chronic pulmonary artery hypertension. *Anesthesiology.* 1992;78:1028–1035.

29. Snow DJ, Gray SJ, Ghosh S, et al. Inhaled nitric oxide in patients with normal and increased pulmonary vascular resistance after cardiac surgery. *Br J Anesth.* 1994;72:185–189.

30. De Wet CJ, Affleck DG, Jacobsohn E, Avidan MS, Tymkew H, Hill LL. Inhaled prostacyclin is safe effective and affordable in patients with pulmonary hypertension, right heart dysfunction, and refractory hypoxemia after cardiothoracic surgery. *J Thor Cardio Surg.* 2004;127:1058–1067.

31. Olshwescki H, Ghofrani HA, Schmehl T, et al. Inhaled illoprost for pulmonary hypertension. *N Eng J Med.* 2002;347(5):322–329.

32. Ghofrani HA, Wiedemann R, Rose F, et al. Combination therapy with oral sildenafil and inhaled iloprost for severe pulmonary hypertension. *Ann Intern Med.* 2002;136(7):515–522.

33. Channick RN, Simonaeu G, Sitbon O, et al. (2001) Effects of the dual endothelin receptor antagonist bosentan in patients with pulm HT: a randomised placebo controlled study. *Lancet.* 2001;358:1119–1123

34. Michelakis E, Tymchal W, Lien D, Webster L, Hashimoto K, Archer S. Oral sildenafil is an effective and specific pulmonary vasodilator in patients with pulmonary arterial hypertension. Comparison with inhaled nitric oxide. *Circulation.* 2002;105:2378–2403.

35. Henke CA, Hertz M, Gustafon P. Combined bronchoscopy and mucolytic therapy for patients with severe refractory status asthmaticus on mechanical ventilation. A case report and review of the literature. *Crit Care Med.* 1994;22:1880–1883.

36. Millman M, Millman FM, Goldstein IM, Mercandetti AJ. Use of Acetylcysteine in bronchial asthma—another look. *Ann Allergy.* 1985;54:294–296.

37. Lawson D, Saggers BA. NAC and antibiotics in cystic fibrosis. *BMJ.* 1965;317.

16
Bronchoscopy in the Intensive Care Unit

David F. Treacher

Abstract Fibre-optic bronchoscopy (FOB) is a relatively safe and potentially lifesaving procedure in intubated patients and should be available at all times in the intensive care unit (ICU). In this chapter, the diagnostic and therapeutic indications, relative contraindications, practical aspects of performing bronchoscopy in the ICU, post-bronchoscopy care and training requirements are discussed.

Introduction

Bronchoscopy is the endoscopic examination of the upper airway and tracheo-bronchial tree, and may be performed using either a rigid or flexible fibre-optic instrument. Rigid bronchoscopy is now rarely performed in ICU, but it may still be necessary for major haemoptysis, biopsy of a potentially vascular tumour, foreign body removal and the placement of airway stents. Fibre-optic bronchoscopy (FOB), however, is indicated for a wide range of diagnostic and therapeutic purposes and can be lifesaving: all ICUs should have rapid access to an instrument and a suitably trained operator should be available on site.[1] Most critically ill patients in whom bronchoscopy is indicated will either be endotracheally intubated or have a tracheostomy in situ. If not, the inspired oxygen concentration that the patient requires, the potential detrimental impact of sedation and having an unprotected airway will usually make it prudent to intubate the patient, at least for the procedure. The remainder of this chapter focuses on FOB and assumes that the patient has a protected airway.

Indications

Although fibre-optic bronchoscopy (FOB) is relatively safe when performed by an experienced operator, patients in ICU are at higher risk of complications[1] and the following question should always be asked: 'Is it indicated, what will it achieve, and what could the complications be?'

Table 16.1 shows the main diagnostic and therapeutic indications.

Diagnostic

Most patients with pneumonia or diffuse alveolar shadowing will initially be managed by obtaining a non-bronchoscopic lavage (NBL) specimen for culture. Bronchoscopy is only indicated to obtain a broncho-alveolar lavage (BAL) or a protected specimen brush (PSB) specimen when there is no persuasive microbiology from the NBL, in the immuno-compromised or HIV-positive patient, when a true alveolar specimen for a cell count is required, to assess the presence of endobronchial Kaposi's sarcoma or if a transbronchial biopsy is indicated. To perform a BAL the bronchoscope should be wedged in the relevant lung segment, 60–80 mL of sterile saline is instilled with the suction switched off and, after waiting for two inspirations, low suction is reintroduced to obtain a 'drizzle' aspirate, the first part of which is discarded. Properly performed BAL has been shown to have a sensitivity of 53–93% and a specificity of 60–95% in diagnosing ventilator-associated pneumonia. BAL can also significantly improve the diagnosis in cases of sputum smear-negative

TABLE 16.1. Indications for bronchoscopy

Diagnostic
- Alveolar infiltrates/ atypical pneumonia
- Transbronchial biopsy
- Haemoptysis
- Thermal or chemical injury
- Blunt chest trauma
- Intubation damage
- Persistent cough
- Post lung transplantation or lung resection

Therapeutic
- Endobronchial intubation
- Excessive thick secretions
- Persistent lobar collapse
- Haemoptysis—localisation and control
- Massive aspiration and removal of foreign body
- Percutaneous tracheostomy

tuberculosis, invasive aspergillosis, coccidiodomy-cosis, cryptococcosis and viral pneumonia.[2] The value of protected specimen brush (PSB) and quantitative bacterial cultures in distinguishing between colonisation and infection remains contentious but may reduce mortality from ventilator-associated pneumonia.[3] Transbronchial biopsy may be indicated for histological diagnosis in the context of diffuse alveolar infiltrates, particularly when an active fibrotic process is suspected and steroid therapy is being considered, but there is the risk of pneumothorax (~10%) and haemorrhage (~5%) and the yield is less than 50%.[4,5] If available, open lung biopsy is preferred as it too can be performed on the unit, has a higher yield and carries less risk.

When performed for haemoptysis, the intention should be to diagnose and localise the source of bleeding, which includes suction catheter trauma, endotracheal tube granulation tissue, tumour, bronchiectasis, TB cavity and pneumonia.

Following thermal or chemical injury to the lungs, which can occur despite the absence of any externally apparent damage, bronchoscopy enables early diagnosis of the anatomical extent and severity of the mucosal erythema, oedema, necrosis and sloughing and allows toilet of obstructing debris.

Bronchoscopy is indicated to assess endobronchial damage after blunt chest trauma, such as steering wheel injuries, particularly in the presence of haemoptysis, surgical emphysema, a flail segment or chest x-ray (CXR) appearances of mediastinal emphysema, segmental collapse or

pneumo/haemothorax. The damage that may be identified ranges from bronchial contusion or rupture, particularly affecting the RUL, to complete tracheal transection. Bronchial disruption requires urgent surgical intervention and therefore early diagnosis is necessary.

Upper airway trauma, related to the procedure of endotracheal intubation itself, may occur early or present later as laryngeal/glottic oedema or formation of granulation tissue. This latter problem is often due to recurrent trauma from the distal tip of the tube, and may be identified by withdrawing the tube over the bronchoscope up to the level of the cords. While the bronchoscope can prevent soiling from limited pharyngeal secretions during this procedure it cannot deal with massive aspiration and so the patient must be nil by mouth for at least 4 h for this elective procedure.

Inspection of the bronchial stump following lung transplant or resection allows identification of an anastomotic air leak, leak from the bronchial suture line, bleeding from suture granuloma or persistent cough caused by an endobronchial suture.[6]

Therapeutic

With the endotracheal tube slipped over a fibreoptic bronchoscope it can be used to guide endotracheal intubation in patients with epiglottitis, laryngeal oedema, tetanus with trismus, trauma to the upper airway and cervical spine injury or deformity such as ankylosing spondylitis. At the same time correct positioning of the endotracheal tube can be confirmed and abnormalities that may be causing gas exchange problems identified. In these situations it is advisable to attempt the bronchoscopic intubation in an operating theatre with an ENT surgeon available to perform an emergency tracheostomy if necessary.

Patients with excessive secretions, not cleared by routine suctioning and physiotherapy, who develop hypoxaemia and/or CXR changes may benefit from bronchoscopy when thick, tenacious secretions occluding a major lobar orifice may be removed by suctioning or following direct instillation of acetylcysteine.

Lobar collapse that has not responded to physiotherapy, and which may be due to retained thick secretions, can be effectively treated by bronchoscopy with locally directed suction and saline or acetylcysteine lavage.[7] Acetylcysteine can cause bronchospasm and the patient should receive a nebulised inhaled bronchodilator prophylactically. Retained secretions should also be considered

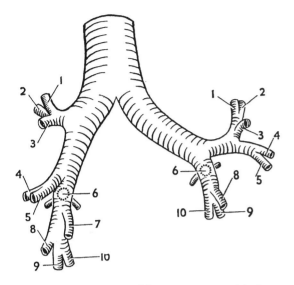

FIGURE 16.1. Anterior view of the major segments of the bronchial tree. 1, 2, 3—Apical, posterior and anterior segments of the upper lobes. 4, 5—Lateral and medial segments of middle lobe on right and superior and inferior segments of lingula on left. 6, 7, 8, 9, 10—Apical, medial basal (right side only), anterior basal, lateral basal and posterior basal segments of lower lobes.

when there is failure of re-expansion of a pneumothorax with persisting air leak despite appropriate positioning of a chest drain. Persisting right upper lobe collapse will occasionally prove to be due to a malpositioned endotracheal tube, with the distal end lying beyond the RUL orifice. This should of course be easily identified on the CXR.

It may be possible to deal with minor haemoptysis caused by suction catheter or endotracheal tube trauma with the use of cold saline or topical vasoconstrictors (epinephrine 1:10,000 solution), and to perform toilet to remove blood from the bronchial tree (Figure 16.1). However, if there has been a major haemoptysis and active bleeding has ceased and a fresh clot is seen in a major bronchus, the temptation to apply suction to it should be resisted since further major uncontrollable haemoptysis may ensue (Figure 16.2). Major haemoptysis (>300 mL over 24h) may be controlled by endobronchial balloon tamponade, using a Fogarty catheter passed down beside the bronchoscope and advanced into the relevant bronchial orifice. The catheter is then inflated and left in situ after withdrawal of the bronchoscope. If the bleeding cannot be controlled to allow localisation of the source, rigid bronchoscopy is indicated. Fibrin glue has also been used to seal the culprit bronchus and if successful this has the advantage that

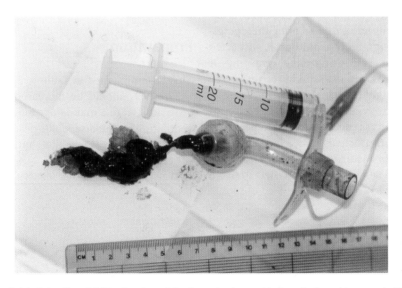

FIGURE 16.2. Blood clot obstructing distal tracheostomy tube, lower trachea and both major bronchi removed with a bronchoscope The bronchoscope, with a new tracheostomy tube mounted on it, was then passed through the tracheal stoma into the trachea thereby allowing re-intubation of the patient and further bronchial toilet.

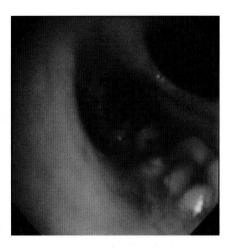

FIGURE 16.3. Cobblestone appearance of endobronchial aspergillosis in the right upper lobe of a patient with systemic lupus erythematosis

TABLE 16.2. Relative contraindications to bronchoscopy in the ICU patient

• Patients requiring high levels of FIO_2 and/or PEEP
• Coagulopathy
• Platelets <50,000 × 10^9/mL
• Severe asthma
• Creatinine >300 µmol/L
• Acute coronary syndrome
• Life-threatening arrhythmia
• SVC obstruction

it dissolves after about 8 days, preventing permanent blockage and the development of bronchiectasis.[8] With the site identified the patient should be nursed with this side dependent, so that further bleeding can only soil one lung, while arrangements are made for therapeutic intervention by embolisation or possibly, and if available, lung resection (Figure 16.3).

Following massive aspiration early bronchoscopy is indicated to remove food debris but it has little role in gastric acid aspiration where it will merely confirm erythema of the proximal bronchial tree but will have little to offer therapeutically. Where foreign body aspiration is suspected (tooth, pea, etc.), FOB using either grasping or basket forceps may be successful in retrieving the item but if not rigid bronchoscopy is indicated.

For the relatively inexperienced operator or whenever difficulty is encountered when performing a percutaneous tracheostomy, a bronchoscope should be used to ensure midline puncture of the trachea and to deal with airway problems related to bleeding or tracheal damage.

Contraindications

These are listed in Table 16.2. Since bronchoscopy can be lifesaving these are only relative contraindications based on a balance of potential risk and benefit. For example, severe hypoxemia to exclude

mucus plugging is quite a common indication for bronchoscopy, therefore high levels of FiO_2 and positive end-expiratory pressure (PEEP) are only relative contraindications but warrant a speedy examination with interruptions as necessary during which the bronchoscope is withdrawn to allow 'bagging' with 100% oxygen. Platelets should be >50 × 10^9 or in the presence of active bleeding >100 × 10^9/mL and coagulation corrected to an INR and APTTR <1.4. Patients with renal failure in whom urgent bronchoscopy is indicated should be given the vasopressin analogue DDAVP.[9] Asthmatic patients should be pretreated with a nebulised bronchodilator and saline warmed to body temperature should be used for any lavage procedures. Glycopyrrolate should be drawn up ready for administration in patients in whom there is a history of vagal sensitivity such as marked bradycardia on suctioning.

Preparation

This is summarised in Table 16.3

The FiO_2 should be increased to 1.0 and the ventilator set to a mandatory mode to ensure that ventilation remains adequate despite sedation and the increased resistance due to the obstruction of

TABLE 16.3. Preparation for bronchoscopy

• Check INR, APTTR, platelets
• Review CXR
• Consider patient co-morbidities
• Monitor ECG and SpO_2
• Set ventilator to back-up mandatory mode
• Increase FIO2 to 1.0
• Give nebulised bronchodilator if asthma history or planning to give acetylcysteine
• Insert mouth guard to prevent damage to bronchoscope
• Sedate and if necessary paralyse the patient

the airway by the bronchoscope. If an infusion of a sedative agent such as propofol and an opiate infusion such as fentanyl are already being administered, the rate can be increased but otherwise a bolus of fentanyl and either propofol or a benzodiazepine such as midazolam can be given. Topical anaesthesia up to a maximum of 15 mL 1% lidocaine can be administered and will help to suppress cough. If despite these measures, the patient continues to cough or bite on the tube, a short-acting muscle relaxant is indicated.

Head-injured patients require profound anaesthesia with neuromuscular blockade to prevent marked rises in intracranial pressure.

Performance

The closed suction unit should be replaced with a catheter mount featuring a swivel adaptor and flexible diaphragm that will admit the bronchoscope, but provide an airtight seal. A bronchoscope with a wide suction channel, up to 3.2 mm diameter, will usually be selected to allow aspiration of thick tenacious secretions. This will have an external diameter of 5.9 mm and occupy 44%, 55% and over 70% of the lumen of tubes sized 9, 8 and 7, respectively, and explains why a tube of at least 8 mm internal diameter is preferred to prevent inadequate ventilation of the patient and damage to the bronchoscope. Generous lubrication of the bronchoscope also helps to prevent damage and aids manoeuvrability of the scope. If the patient has a smaller tube and it is considered unsafe to change it, a paediatric scope can be used, but this essentially limits the investigation to the diagnostic options.

An assistant, usually the bedside nurse, should support the tube during the procedure, insert the traps to collect specimens and observe the oxygen saturation, tidal volume and other vital signs. They should alert the operator to the problems that may require temporary interruption of the procedure. During the procedure the use and level of suction must not be excessive to prevent mucosal damage and the loss of PEEP causing de-recruitment and hypoxaemia. The procedure should be thorough, with inspection of all 20 bronchial segments, collection of the necessary specimens and performance of appropriate toilet. However, inappropriate delays should be avoided as they increase the risks of the procedure for the patient.

Complications

When performed by a suitably trained operator bronchoscopy in the intubated patient is a safe procedure. Many of the complications are predictable and the decision should be made either not to perform the procedure or to take the necessary precautions to deal with cardiac arrest and dysrhythmias in the patient with a cardiac history or bronchospasm in known asthmatics. Some degree of oxygen desaturation and carbon dioxide retention are almost inevitable, particularly in patients with acute lung injury on high levels of PEEP. After a CXR has been performed to exclude a pneumothorax, a recruitment manoeuvre will usually improve oxygenation.

A fever is quite common (~15%) after bronchoscopy and an episode of ventilator-associated pneumonia may occur but is less likely if the procedure is brief and excessive lavage of the bronchial segments is avoided.[10]

Post-bronchoscopy Care

Following bronchoscopy, the ventilator settings should be returned towards the previously set levels after ensuring that the patient has recovered from the sedation and paralysis. The FiO_2 should be reduced according to the arterial oxygen saturation and blood gases. A CXR should be performed if a biopsy has been taken, if there were complications during the procedure or if the patient becomes unstable following the procedure.

Complete details of the procedure should be recorded, preferably on a standardised sheet or on a computer to allow audit to be easily performed. The patient name and bronchoscope number should be identified in the report so that any infection control issues can be investigated.

The scope should be cleaned post procedure by the operator to ensure that secretions, which may permanently damage the scope, are removed from the suction channel by thorough flushing with saline. The bronchoscope should then be returned to the infection control unit for disinfection.

Training

Before being considered competent to perform a bronchoscopy in ICU, the trainee should be able to describe the procedure to the patient/relative and obtain consent/assent, give appropriate sedation/paralysis to the patient, maintain the airway and adequate oxygenation, identify all the main segmental bronchi, perform bronchial brushing and lavage and manage the complications of tenacious secretions, haemorrhage, hypoxaemia and pneumothorax.[11] Most bronchoscope systems now have the image displayed on a video screen, which makes the demonstration of the bronchial segments and the various manoeuvres much easier. Most trainees are competent to perform an unsupervised bronchoscopy, albeit with assistance available, after being directed for ten procedures.

References

1. BTS Guidelines Committee. British Thoracic Society Guidelines on Diagnostic Flexible Bronchoscopy. *Thorax*. 2001;56i:12–14.
2. Jolliet P, Chevrolet JC. Bronchoscopy in the ICU. *Intensive Care Med*. 1992;18:160.
3. Fagon JY, Chastre J, Wolff M, et al. Invasive and non-invasive strategies for management of suspected ventilator-associated pneumonia: a randomized trial. *Ann Intern Med*. 2000;132:621–630.
4. Pincus PS, Kallenbach JM, Hurwitz MD, Clinton C, Feldman C, Abramowitz JA, et al. Transbronchial biopsy during mechanical ventilation. *Crit Care Med*. 1987;15:1136.
5. O'Brien JD, Ettinger NA, Shevlin D, Kollef MH. Safety and yield of transbronchial biopsy in mechanically ventilated patients. *Crit Care Med*. 1997;25:440–446.
6. Albertini RE. Cough caused by endobronchial sutures. *Ann Intern Med*. 1981;94:205.
7. Marini JJ, Pierson DJ, Hudson LD. Acute lobar atelectasis: a prospective comparison of fibreoptic bronchoscopy and respiratory therapy. *Am Rev Respir Dis*. 1979;119:971.
8. Matar AF, Hill JH, Duncan W, Orfanakis N, Law I. Use of biological glue to control pulmonary air leaks. *Thorax*. 1990;46:670.
9. Kobrinsky NL, Cheang MS, Gerrard JM, et al. Shortening of bleeding time by 1-deamino-8-D-arginine vasopressin in various bleeding disorders. *Lancet*. 1984;2:1145.
10. Pereira W, Kovnat DM, Khan MA, Iacovino JR, Spivack ML, Snider GL. Fever and pneumonia after flexible fibreoptic bronchoscopy. *Am Rev Respir Dis*. 1975;112:59.
11. Bone RC, Aviles A, Faber LP. Guidelines for competency and training in fiberoptic bronchoscopy. *Chest*. 1982;81:739.

17
Tracheostomy and Mini-Tracheostomy

Ulrike Buehner and Andy Bodenham

Abstract Percutaneous dilational tracheostomy (PDT) is currently accepted as the standard technique for longer-term airway management in the critically ill patient in many intensive care units (ICUs). This chapter gives an overview of applied anatomy and techniques, answering the questions of timing, indications, complications, choice of tracheostomy tube and post-tracheostomy care.

Introduction

Open surgical tracheostomy is one of the oldest surgical procedures. It was first formalised in 1909 by Chevalier Jackson.[1] In 1985, Ciaglia and colleagues introduced the percutaneous dilatational tracheostomy (PDT) technique: a bedside procedure involving the insertion of a tracheostomy tube with minimal dissection through the smallest incision possible.[2] It has since become a popular procedure in ICUs worldwide and is increasingly replacing the surgical technique in critically ill patients.

Indications for Tracheostomy in the ICU

Tracheostomy formation may be indicated in the following circumstances:

- To aid weaning from assisted ventilation and sedation
- Provide tracheal access to remove pulmonary secretions
- Permit long-term airway management
- Bypass upper airway obstruction (e.g. patients with trauma, infection, malignancy, laryngeal or subcricoid stenosis, bilateral recurrent laryngeal nerve palsy)
- Prevent pulmonary aspiration (e.g. patients with laryngeal incompetence: CVA, Parkinson's disease)
- Neuromuscular disorders (e.g. motor neurone disease, critical illness neuromyopathy)
- Bulbar dysfunction
- Severe brain injury

Benefits of Tracheostomy

- Better mouth care
- Allows oral nutrition and earlier mobilisation of patients[3]
- Reduces the need for sedative or analgesic drugs $\rightarrow$ more effective cough and better cooperation with physiotherapy
- Reduces frequency of accidental extubation and endobronchial intubation
- Reduces complications of long-term translaryngeal intubation (e.g. laryngeal damage, subglottic stenosis)
- Lower airway resistance, smaller deadspace, reduced work of breathing $\rightarrow$ improved weaning from assisted ventilation
- Fenestrated tracheostomy tube or cuff deflation allows phonation and better communication
- Earlier discharge from the ICU to a high dependency unit (HDU) or suitable ward

Relative Contraindications to PDT

- Children <12 years old
- Uncorrectable coagulopathy
- Active infection over the anterior neck
- Local malignancy in the trachea
- Unstable cervical spine fracture
- Morbid obesity (BMI > 35)[5-7]
- Gross anatomical distortion of the neck
- Previous neck surgery or tracheostomy[6,7]
- Previous radiotherapy to the neck
- Extensive burns to the neck
- Requirement of high PEEP (>15 cmH$_2$O) or FiO$_2$ (>0.6)
- Haemodynamic instability
- Patients unlikely to survive >48 h

BMI   Body mass index
PEEP   Positive end-expiratory pressure
FiO$_2$ Fraction of inspired oxygen

The list of relative contraindications for PDT may reduce with increasing experience of the operator, use of endoscopy and ultrasound or other imaging of the neck.

Timing

The timing of tracheostomy in critical care is controversial,[10] and data from randomised-controlled trials are scarce.[11-13] The popularity of PDT has resulted in earlier tracheostomies. It has been suggested that early tracheostomy may shorten the length of ICU stay and decrease the incidence of nosocomial pneumonias. A randomised UK-controlled multi-centre trial, 'Tracheostomy management in critical care' (Tracman, www.tracman.org.uk) is currently investigating the potential benefits of early tracheostomy (days 1–4 post-ICU admission) versus late (day 10 or later post-ICU admission).

General Considerations

Two trained operators are required: one with competence in tracheostomy and management of complications and the other in providing general anaesthesia and airway maintenance. The procedure should ideally be performed during normal working hours to ensure the supervision and support from senior staff members and other specialists.

Ultrasound scanning of the neck prior to percutaneous tracheostomy allows visualisation of the anatomy of the anterior neck structures, particularly the assessment of blood vessels and depth and angulation of the trachea. Useful information about adjacent structures helps with the risk–benefit analysis of an open versus percutaneous tracheostomy. Imaging can guide needles and dilators away from at-risk structures.[7]

Endoscopy, using a fibre-optic scope passed through the tracheal tube, may be used to guide correct placement of needle, guidewire and tube. Direct visualisation reduces posterior tracheal wall damage and tube misplacement. However, the presence of a flexible fibre-optic scope may hinder ventilation, increasing the risk of hypoxia and hypercarbia with associated increase in intracranial pressure in susceptible patients. An alternative approach includes the use of metal-cased semi-rigid, small-diameter scopes, such as a Bonfils laryngoscope or optical stylet, which interferes less with ventilation and avoids expensive damage to a flexible scope by needle puncture.

Techniques

The majority of modern percutaneous tracheostomy kits are based on a Seldinger technique using flexible guidewires, plastic introducers and flexible tracheostomy tubes (Figure 17.1).

In 1985, Ciaglia and colleagues introduced the first widely used technique of PDT using a series of dilators of increasing diameter to create a tracheal stoma.[2]

The inward force produced during dilatation of the tracheal wall has been associated with posterior tracheal wall tears and fracture of the tracheal rings. In an attempt to streamline the technique of PDT, the single-step dilator was recently introduced (Blue Rhino kit by Cook and a similar kit by others) with the following advantages:

- The single dilator has a hydrophilic coating, which, when wet, reduces friction and thus allows smooth dilatation of the tracheal stoma. This is quicker and less traumatic.
- Faster technique reduces time during which dilators and bronchoscope obstruct the airway, reducing the risk of hypercarbia and hypoxia.
- The single-step dilator is flexible, tapering to a

FIGURE 17.1. A modern percutaneous tracheostomy kit.

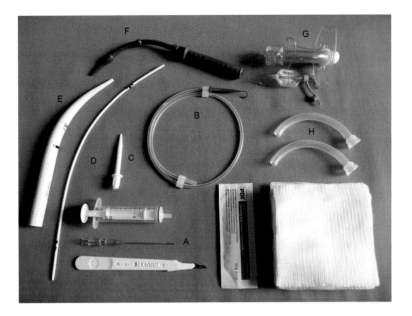

soft malleable tip, which will bend at the required angle to follow the direction of the guidewire down the trachea.

- It avoids the aerolisation of blood in between dilatator changes. The continuous tamponade effect reduces bleeding.

Other techniques currently under evaluation include dilatation with angioplasty-type balloon catheters or other plastic dilators.

The most popular one-step dilatational technique is described here:

1. Full monitoring is ensured (BP, ECG, pulse oximeter and capnography). Anaesthesia includes an intravenous opioid, hypnotic and short-acting muscle relaxant. The ventilator is set to an FiO_2 of 1.0 and volumes are adjusted to compensate for the presence of the bronchoscope and any air leak.

2. The patient is positioned with the head extended by pushing the pillow under the shoulders. This brings as much of the trachea as possible into the neck. From the cricoid cartilage, moving caudally, the tracheal rings are identified (Figure 17.2). The skin is prepared with antiseptic solution and the neck draped to maintain a sterile field. The area of incision is infiltrated with 10–20 mL of local anaesthetic (e.g. lidocaine 1% with epinephrine 1:200,000).

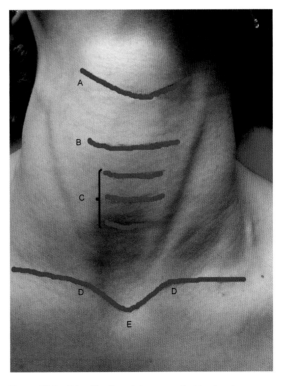

FIGURE 17.2. Identification of the anatomical landmarks
A—Thyroid cartilage
B—Cricoid cartilage
C—First to third tracheal rings
D—Clavicle
E—Sternal notch

A 14 G introducer needle with cannula is inserted into the trachea midline between the second and third tracheal rings under direct endoscopic visualisation. Care is taken to avoid the posterior tracheal wall. Correct needle position may also be confirmed by aspiration of air from the trachea, aspiration of respiratory secretions or capnography.

3. The needle is then removed and a J-tipped guidewire threaded through the cannula into the trachea to the level of the carina. The sheath is removed and replaced by a 14F short dilator which is advanced over the guidewire to dilate the initial access site. Some compression to the anterior tracheal wall is expected. The dilator is removed and replaced by an 8F guiding catheter that is advanced over the guidewire. The guiding catheter and wire are inserted as a unit into the trachea until the safety ridge on the guiding catheter is at skin level. Correct positioning can be confirmed by aligning the proximal end of the catheter with the proximal mark on the guidewire. This will prevent displacement of the J-wire and possible trauma to the posterior tracheal wall during subsequent manipulations. A skin-deep small incision on either side of this assembly is made just big enough to allow passage of the larger dilator.

4. Lubrication is accomplished by dipping the dilator tip into sterile water or saline. This activates its hydrophilic coating. The dilator is held like a pencil and advanced in a curved arching motion until the 39Fr mark reaches the skin. Repeated advancement and retraction of the dilating assembly effectively dilates the tracheal access site. Finally, after verifying its integrity, the well-lubricated tracheostomy tube, preloaded onto a dilator of the appropriate size, is advanced over the guidewire and guiding catheter into the tracheal lumen. The latter two are removed, leaving the tracheostomy tube in place. The cuff is inflated with air until no air leak is heard. The cuff pressure should not exceed $25\,cmH_2O$ (18 mmHg). It is important that this is checked regularly to prevent complications of tracheal mucosal damage, stenosis and tracheo-oesophageal fistula. Ventilation is confirmed by capnography, bilateral chest movement and auscultation.

5. The tube may need suctioning to clear any residual blood clots and secretions formed during the procedure. The tube should be tied in securely. A fibre-optic scope can be used to inspect the trachea for trauma and bleeding and to measure the distance from the tube tip to the carina. It can also be passed from above through the glottis to assess the adequacy of the position and length of the tracheostomy tube. Some tubes will be seen to be too short with the cuff being pulled up against the anterior tracheal wall. In this case the tube should be exchanged for a longer adjustable flange tube. A portable chest radiograph will rule out other complications, such as pneumothorax or subcutaneous emphysema, but is not essential in the routine case.

Complications

Perioperative

- Bleeding
- Puncture of the endotracheal (ET) tube cuff
- Needle damage to the fibre-optic bronchoscope
- Dislodgement of the ET tube
- Anaesthetic awareness
- Hypoxia
- Hypercapnia
- Increased intracranial pressure
- Damage to the trachea
- Damage to the oesophagus
- False passage of tracheostomy tube
- Pneumothorax/pneumomediastinum
- Airway obstruction due to blood clot

Postoperative
Early

- Collapsed lung
- Surgical emphysema
- Dislodgement of the tracheostomy tube
- Airway obstruction due to blood clot
- Tension pneumothorax

Late

- Bleeding (e.g. erosion into innominate artery/vein)
- Local stomal infection
- Subglottic/tracheal stenosis
- Tracheo-oesophageal fistula
- Persistent trachea to skin fistula
- Scarring and tethering of the trachea

Complications of PDT, including bleeding, infection and hypoxia, are infrequent. Most are minor with no serious sequelae. Minor bleeding and puncture of the endotracheal (ET) tube cuff are the most common complications. However, when complications do occur, they can be devastating. There is a risk of damage to the trachea, including rupture and displacement of the tracheal rings, tear of the posterior tracheal wall and tracheo-oesophageal fistula. All of these may be associated with bleeding, and the formation of false passages as well as major air leaks.

There are now a number of publications showing that PDT is associated with a lower incidence of perioperative and early postoperative complications compared with open surgical tracheostomy. Friedman and colleagues randomised 26 patients to receive PDT and 27 patients to receive an open tracheostomy performed in the operating theatre.[8] There was no difference in perioperative complications (transient hypertension, hypoxia, subcutaneous emphysema, small bleed and loss of airway). The number of post-procedural complications was significantly higher in the surgical tracheostomy group (41%) than in the PDT group (12%), predominantly as a result of wound or stomal infection and accidental decannulation. Freeman and co-workers compiled data from five prospective controlled studies (236 patients) and found no difference between PDT and surgical tracheostomy in overall operative complications and mortality.[9] The overall postoperative complication rate of PDT was lower particularly regarding the incidence of bleeding and infection.

Choice of Tracheostomy Tube

There is a wide range of tubes commercially available:

- Rigid versus flexible
- Plain versus cuffed (profile versus non-profile cuff)
- Non-crease cuffs
- Fixed length versus adjustable flange
- Inner liner for ease of cleaning
- Fenestrations for communication
- PVC/silver/silastic materials

- Flexible, metallic-reinforced tubes for distorted airway anatomy
- Additional suction channels to remove secretions

Soft and flexible tubes provide maximum patient comfort, minimising any trauma to the trachea and associated structures (Figures 17.3 and 17.4). Rigid tubes are used more commonly in the longer term as they are thought to keep the stoma open better and are easier to change. Cuffed tubes provide airway protection and facilitate intermittent positive pressure ventilation. Disadvantages include the risk of excessive cuff pressure and difficulty in swallowing and communication. High-volume low-pressure cuffs reduce the incidence of cuff-related mucosal damage by providing a wider surface area of the trachea for the pressure to be dissipated. Newer cuffs, which have no folds or creases and are claimed to avoid microaspiration are also available.

Adjustable flange tubes are designed for patients whose trachea is deeper than usual below the skin and soft tissues in the neck, e.g. obese patients.

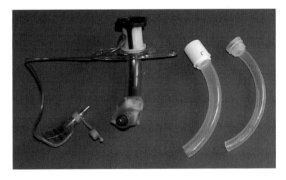

FIGURE 17.3. An example of a soft and flexible tracheostomy.

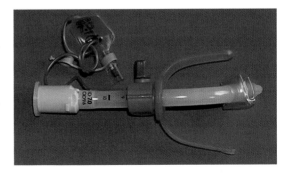

FIGURE 17.4. A soft, flexible tracheostomy tube featuring an adjustable flange.

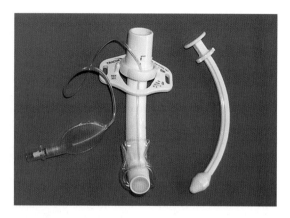

FIGURE 17.5.   A rigid tracheostomy tube with inner cannula in situ and obturator.

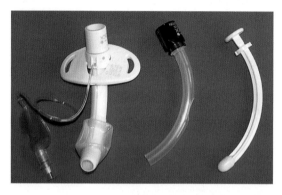

FIGURE 17.6.   A rigid, fenestrated tracheostomy tube with inner fenestrated and non-fenestrated cannulae plus obturator.

Tracheostomy tubes with an inner tube may remain in place up to 30 days or more as the inner cannula can be cleaned and changed regularly (Figure 17.5). A disadvantage is that the diameter of the inner lumen will be reduced by 1–2 mm, increasing work of breathing.

A fenestrated tube allows airflow through the vocal cords when the tube is occluded or a speaking valve is attached (Figure 17.6). It is unsuitable for patients fully dependent on positive pressure ventilation unless a non-fenestrated inner cannula is used and increases the potential for aspiration of gastric contents.

Role of Minitracheostomy

A small-diameter (4 mm ID), uncuffed tube can be inserted percutaneously via the cricothyroid membrane following infiltration with local anaesthetic. This facilitates treatment of sputum retention by providing access for regular suction of respiratory secretions. This technique has also been used in the emergency management of upper airway obstruction.

Limitations of the mintracheostomy kit include small-bore suction and inability to provide continuous positive airway pressure (CPAP) or positive pressure ventilation. There is no cuff for airway protection.

Aftercare

Adequate humidification, tracheal suctioning and physiotherapy are essential to avoid obstruction of tracheostomy tubes. For those with inner tubes, regular removal for cleaning is important to maintain tube patency. Tubes without inner cannulae should be exchanged every 10–14 days.

A tracheostomy tube blocked with tenacious secretions renders the patient at risk of progressive hypoxia and possibly cardiorespiratory arrest.

Resuscitation attempts will be unsuccessful unless the airway obstruction is recognised and treated promptly. Removal of the tracheostomy tube may be required if suctioning fails to clear the obstruction. In the short term, spontaneously breathing patients will usually manage to breathe through their own airway. If the tracheostomy is more than 1 week old, the stoma is generally well established to allow early tube replacement if required.

For patients dependent on assisted ventilation, re-intubation by the oral route may be needed in the interim if difficulties occur in replacing the tracheostomy tube.

When caring for a tracheostomy patient, the following equipment should always remain with the patient:

- Tracheostomy tubes (same size as in situ plus one size smaller)
- Tracheal dilators
- Suction unit, catheters and gloves
- Self-inflating bag-valve mask device and tubing
- A 10 mL syringe for cuff de/inflation
- Translaryngeal intubation equipment

Decannulation

Decannulation should be considered when patients demonstrate a satisfactory respiratory drive, a good cough and the ability to protect their own airway. Patients who show no signs of tiring on continuous positive airway pressure (CPAP) or a T-piece with low flow oxygen therapy are candidates for decannulation. Coughing secretions up into the tracheostomy tube is a good sign whereas generalised weakness and inability to hold the head up are negative predictors of successful decannulation. An impaired conscious level also reduces the chance of success.

Tracheostomy tubes should be removed as soon as feasible to regain the normal physiological functions of active coughing, upper airway warming, humidification and filtering of air.

Following decannulation, most tracheostomy stomas are allowed to granulate without suturing. They achieve a functional seal within 2–3 days. These partially healed wounds can be quickly reopened with an artery forceps in the first few weeks after closure if necessary.[7] Occasional patients will require ENT referral for tracheal stenosis, tethered scars or a persistent sinus from skin to trachea.

References

1. Jackson C. Tracheostomy. Laryngoscope. 1909;19: 285–290.
2. Ciaglia P, Firsching R, Syniec C. Elective percutaneous dilatational tracheostomy. *Chest*. 1985;87: 715–719.
3. Plummer AL, Gracy DR. Consensus conference on artificial airways in patients receiving mechanical ventilation. *Chest*. 1989;96:178–180.
4. Barry B, Bodenham AR. The role of tracheostomy in ICU. *Anaesth Intensive Care Med*. 2004;11:375–378.
5. Mansharamani NG, Koziel H, Garland R, LoCicero J 3rd, Critchlow J, Ernst A. Safety of beside percutaneous dilatational tracheostomy in obese patients in the ICU. *Chest*. 2000;117:1426–1429.
6. Meyer M, Critchlow J, Mansharamani NG, Angel LF, Garland R, Ernst A. Repeat bedside percutaneous dilatational tracheostomy is a safe procedure. *Crit Care Med*. 2002;30:986–988.
7. Paw HGW, Bodenham AR (2004). *Percutaneous Tracheostomy: A Practical Handbook*. Cambridge: Greenwich Medical Media; 2004. ISBN 1 84110 142 7.
8. Friedman Y, Fildes J, Mizock B, et al. Comparison of percutaneous and surgical tracheostomies. *Chest*. 1995;110:480–485.
9. Freeman BD, Isabella K, Cobb JP, et al. A prospective, randomised study comparing percutaneous with surgical tracheostomy in critically ill patients. *Crit Care Med*. 2001;29:926–930.
10. Heffner JE. Tracheostomy application and timing. *Clin Chest Med*. 2003;24:389–398.
11. Sugerman HJ, Wolfe L, Pasquale MD, et al. Multicenter, randomised, prospective trial of early tracheostomy. *J Trauma*. 1997;43: 741–747.
12. Saffle JR, Morris SE, Edelman L. Early tracheostomy does not improve outcome in burn patients. *J Burn Care Rehabil*. 2002;23:431–438.
13. Rumbale MJ, Newton M, Truncale T, et al. A Prospective, randomised, study comparing early percutaneous dilational tracheotomy to prolonged translaryngeal intubation (delayed tracheotomy) in critically ill medical patients. *Crit Care Med*. 2004; 32:1689–1694.

18
Weaning from Mechanical Ventilation

Nicholas Hart

Abstract Weaning from mechanical ventilation can be a complex and difficult task and has generated increased attention over the past few years, particularly in relation to the definitions of weaning delay and failure. In addition, our understanding of the pathophysiology of weaning has been enhanced through the development of the respiratory muscle load-capacity-drive model of weaning failure. A number of randomised, controlled trials have directed clinical practice in terms of the optimal mode of ventilation, as well as assessing the readiness of a patient to wean by incorporating weaning protocols. Although the weaning process has also been improved in patients with chronic respiratory disease, by using non-invasive ventilation at the point of extubation, this practice should not be extended to all patients since there is evidence that it can negatively impact on outcome. Despite a distinct lack of clinical trials, weaning centres appear to have a role in weaning patients with weaning delay and failure. Looking to the future, it is possible that computer-driven automated weaning machines may find a place in our practice; however, evidence is emerging that addressing psychological issues in the patient is also an important factor in shortening the weaning process.

Introduction

Weaning from mechanical ventilation can be one of the most challenging tasks for critical care specialists. It must be considered as two separate processes: the first is liberation from mechanical ventilation, followed by the second phase, extubation or decannulation.

Is Weaning from Mechanical Ventilation a Real Problem?

Around 75% of patients who require invasive ventilatory support can be liberated in less than 10 days from initiation of weaning.[1–3] However, in the remaining 25% weaning is a difficult, expensive[4] and time-consuming task, with 5–10% of patients still requiring ventilatory support at 30 days.[5]

Definition of Weaning Delay and Failure

A Department of Health report 'Weaning and Long-Term Ventilation'[6] has provided workable definitions for both weaning delay and failure. Weaning delay is the need for ventilatory support for more than 14 days in the absence of any non-respiratory factor preventing weaning, whereas weaning failure is defined as ventilator dependence for more than 21 days. Although arbitrary, these definitions provide a framework for critical care specialists and it is useful to classify patients as simple (less than 14 days), difficult (14–21 days) and very difficult (more than 21 days) to wean. Within these definitions, the NHS Modernisation agency identified the point prevalence of weaning delay and failure in the UK as 8% and 7%, respectively.[6]

Pathophysiology of Weaning Failure

Adequate alveolar ventilation is essential to maintain carbon dioxide homeostasis and is determined by the difference between minute and dead space ventilation. By focussing on factors that influence frequency (f) and tidal volume (V_T), the reasons for weaning failure can be better understood. Central drive, neuromuscular transmission, respiratory muscle action and respiratory system impedance are all important and impairment at one or more levels can result in weaning problems (Figure 18.1).

It is important not to consider respiratory muscle drive, load and capacity in isolation, since weaning failure is recognised as an imbalance between all three components (Figure 18.2). A structured approach should be applied in difficult-to-wean

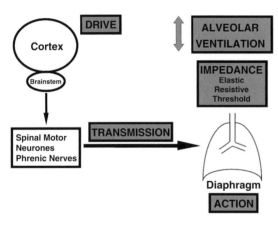

FIGURE 18.1. Factors influencing alveolar ventilation.

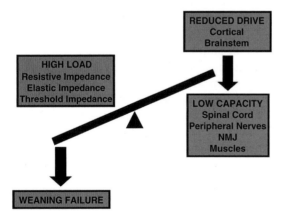

FIGURE 18.2. Respiratory muscle pump: weaning failure as a consequence of an imbalance between respiratory muscle drive, load and capacity.

patients, identifying the clinical conditions implicated in failure of drive and neurotransmission, reduced respiratory muscle performance and increased impedance (Figure 18.3).

Using this approach it is simple to highlight the pathophysiological processes in chronic obstructive airways disease (COPD) (Figure 18.4).

Although this framework for weaning failure is well established in physiological terms, advances in technology have enabled recent studies to examine the influence of pulmonary mechanics, respiratory muscle strength and fatigue on weaning outcome. Whilst studies have shown that COPD patients successfully weaning from mechanical ventilation have lower airways resistance, intrinsic positive end-expiratory pressure (PEEPi) and elastic load at the end of a spontaneous breathing trial compared with those who fail, the elastic, resistive and threshold loads at the start of the trial are similar in both groups.[7] Furthermore, diaphragm strength is similar in patients who successfully wean compared with those who fail and there is, in fact, no evidence of diaphragm fatigue in the failure group at the end of a weaning trial.[8] All these data suggest that deterioration in pulmonary mechanics during a trial of spontaneous ventilation is one of the most important determinants of weaning outcome.

Initiation of Weaning

Weaning should be considered as three distinct phases:

• Assessment of the readiness to wean
• Evaluation of the response to a reduction in ventilatory support
• Extubation or decannulation

Furthermore, weaning should be considered to start at the point when a patient is changed from a controlled to a spontaneous mode of ventilation. Prolonged invasive mechanical ventilation is detrimental to outcome. There is not only an increased risk of nosocomial pneumonia, but also an increased incidence of persistent weaning failure and mortality, especially in patients with COPD.[9–11] Although the goal is to start weaning early, it is essential that attention is focused on difficult-to-wean

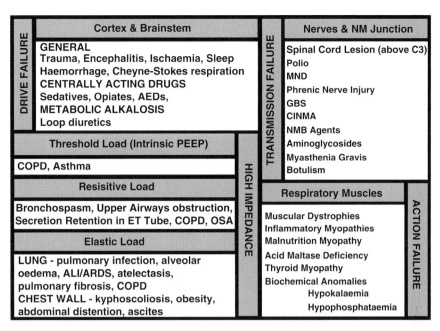

FIGURE 18.3. Causes of weaning failure: drive failure, transmission failure, action failure and high impedance *Abbreviations:* AEDs = anti-epileptic drugs; COPD = chronic obstructive airways disease; ET = endotracheal tube; OSA = obstructive sleep apnoea; ALI/ARDS = acute lung injury/acute respiratory distress syndrome; MND = motor neurone disease; GBS = Guillain–Barré syndrome; CINMA = critical illness neuromuscular abnormality; NMB = neuromuscular blocking agents.

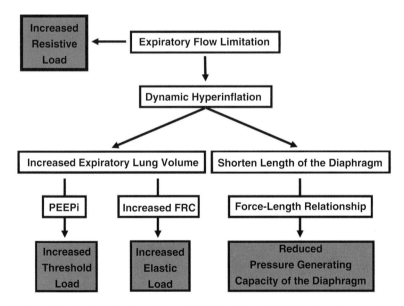

FIGURE 18.4. Pathophysiology of chronic obstructive airways disease (COPD) *Abbreviations:* PEEPi = intrinsic positive end-expiratory pressure and FRC = functional residual capacity.

patients, such as those with COPD, chronic heart failure (CHF) and neuromuscular disease (NMD).[12,13] In these three groups 40–70% of the time spent on mechanical ventilation is during the weaning phase.[13] However, this should not result in a nihilistic approach to COPD patients requiring invasive ventilatory support. Esteban et al.[13] showed that the weaning time in COPD patients was similar to that of CHF patients and, furthermore, the duration of invasive mechanical ventilation is less than that of NMD patients.

Although the aim is to identify difficult-to-wean patients and start weaning early, premature weaning attempts can subject patients to a tenfold increase in work of breathing,[7] which must be viewed as an adverse physiological event in the weaning process. Whilst a failed, planned extubation carries a sixfold increase in mortality,[14,15] only 30% of unplanned extubations during weaning require re-intubation,[15] which could be interpreted as our overcautious approach to weaning and extubation.

Prediction of Successful Weaning

Table 18.1 shows the standard criteria for initiation of weaning. In the last 20 years, there have been over 20 published studies using the frequency/tidal volume (f/V_T) ratio as a predictor of weaning outcome in adult patients. In combination, these studies have recruited in excess of 1,700 patients. However, the results of these studies are conflicting. One of the original studies by Yang and Tobin[16] used a threshold f/V_T ratio of ≤100 breaths/min/L (b/min/L). In this study, the negative predictive value was 0.95 with a positive predictive value of 0.78, that is, the test predicted failure better than success. Review of all the studies reveals a variety of results with a range of f/V_T ratio values. If only the studies that have used f/V_T ratios between 100–105 b/min/L are included, the ranges of negative and positive predictive values are from 0.19 to 1.0 and from 0.60 to 0.94, respectively.

The reason for this wide variability is the failure to acknowledge the effect of pre-test probability; the interpretation of a test result depends on the pre-test probability of a disease.[17] In essence, to have the most gain from a diagnostic test the pre-test probability should be close to 50%, that is, 50% weaning success and 50% weaning failure. However, over half of the studies had weaning success rates of greater than 75%. For a weaning predictor to influence decision making it should be measured early in the course of weaning, when there is 50% pre-test probability, possibly at the point of change from a mandatory to spontaneous mode of ventilation. This explains, in part, the findings of the Weaning Task Force,[18] who identified 462 weaning predictors in 65 observational studies and evaluated the ability of each variable to predict the outcome of a spontaneous breathing trial (SBT). The pooled likelihood ratios of the predictors were all found to have a low predictive power. The task force concluded that weaning predictors should be disregarded and the weaning process initiated with a trial of spontaneous breathing.

The Effect of Ventilatory Mode on Weaning

Following the landmark studies of Brochard et al.[1] and Esteban et al.,[2] synchronised intermittent mandatory ventilation (SIMV) should be disregarded as a mode for effective weaning. The more difficult question to address is whether pressure support ventilation (PSV) or T-piece SBTs is the most favourable mode to successfully wean patients. The study of Brochard and colleagues[1] showed that PSV was better than T-piece SBTs, which was more effective that SIMV. However, Esteban et al.[2] demonstrated that T-piece SBTs was superior to PSV, which showed equivalence with SIMV. The clinical implication from these trials is that it is possible to successfully wean patients using either PSV or T-piece SBTs, but it will depend on the local expertise of the unit as to the mode

TABLE 18.1. General criteria for successful weaning

Neurological	Patient awake and compliant
	Minimal sedative agents required
Respiratory	PaO/FiO$_2$ ≥200 mmHg (FiO$_2$ 0.4)
	f/V_T ≤105 breath/min/L
	PEEP ≤5 cmH$_2$O
	Adequate cough and minimal secretions
Cardiovascular	Haemodynamically stable
	Off vasopressors and ionotropes
Metabolic	Apyrexial
	Hb >8 g/dL (10 g/dL in IHD)
	All electrolytes within normal range

Abbreviations: PaO2 = arterial partial pressure of oxygen; FiO2 = fraction of inspired oxygen; f/VT = frequency to tidal volume ratio; PEEP = positive end-expiratory pressure; IHD = ischaemic heart disease and Hb = haemoglobin.

of ventilation employed. Another interesting issue surrounds the duration of a SBT. Recent data have shown that 30-min SBTs are as effective as 120-min trials in predicting outcome. However, this study involved all patients being considered for weaning and not just those for whom there were difficulties with weaning.[19] These data should therefore be interpreted with caution.

Weaning Protocols

This is another controversial issue. The study by Ely et al.,[5] in common with most of the other weaning studies, compared daily screening and a weaning protocol with physician-led care. The outcome was that the mechanical ventilation time was reduced from 6 to 4 days in the intervention group, but interestingly there was no difference in ICU or hospital stay. Furthermore, although it was emphasised that the cost for the ICU stay was less, there was no difference in the overall cost of treatment between the two groups. There was also a suggestion that more patients in the physician-led group received >21 days of mechanical ventilation, even though patients in this group passed a successful screening test 24 h earlier than the intervention group. This is difficult to explain, but may be a consequence of the weaning mode used in the control group as 76% of these patients were weaned using SIMV, the least preferred mode of weaning from mechanical ventilation.[1,2] Therefore, the main results of this study were that a stepwise approach to weaning with a systematic evaluation of weaning predictors, followed by the assessment of the response to a single T-tube SBT is superior to physician-led care. In fact, close inspection of all of the six published studies assessing the effect of protocol-driven weaning shows that the studies are either flawed in their methodology or that protocols do not improve weaning outcome.[3,5,20–24] Thus, whilst guidelines and protocols have many uses in the ICU, evidence for their role in weaning is limited. This is important for all critical care specialists as weaning should be regarded as a dynamic process that requires an in-depth understanding and application of physiological principles and not a process that can be dictated by an inflexible protocol.

The Role of Non-invasive Ventilation (NIV) Following Weaning and Extubation

There is no controversy surrounding this issue. It has been shown in three randomised controlled trials that NIV is an effective tool to facilitate extubation in patients with chronic respiratory disease and persistent weaning failure.[25–27] In particular, in difficult-to-wean patients with COPD, NIV has been shown to reduce the time of invasive ventilation, shorten ICU and hospital stay, decrease the incidence of nosocomial pneumonia, reduce the need for tracheostomy and improve survival.[25–27] However, the results of these studies should be interpreted with caution as NIV is not applicable to unselected groups of weaning patients. This is highlighted by the recent study of Esteban et al.,[28] which demonstrated that NIV actually increased mortality in patients with post-extubation respiratory distress. But, only 10% of patients in this study had COPD and most of the proven benefit of NIV is in patients with COPD rather than hypoxaemic respiratory failure. Furthermore, in this study there was a delay in re-intubation time in the NIV group, which would have been expected to adversely affect outcome.

Cost and Clinical Effectiveness of Weaning Centres

Although in the UK there are few weaning centres, in North America weaning centres are increasing at an almost alarming rate, raising concern about staff training and quality of care. A significant driver for this increase in weaning centres in the US is financial. It has been estimated that there are over 11,000 ventilator-dependent patients in acute care facilities costing over $9 million a day.[4] In the UK, a point prevalence survey has shown that the incidence of weaning delay and failure in the UK is 8% and 7%, respectively, and it has been estimated that there could be a 50% cost-saving per patient day in managing a tracheostomised ventilator-dependent patient in a level 2 rather than a level 3 facility.[6] In a 1-year study in the North of England by Robson et al[29], these patients were shown to occupy 1,000 bed days in level 3 facilities. If these patients occupied level 2 rather than level 3 beds, a saving of £400,000 could be made.[29] Extrapolation of these data to the whole of England suggests a cost-saving in excess of £5 million per year.[6] However, this calculation can be criticised as a conservative approximation as the estimated cost of level 2 occupancy was £400 per day and that of level 3 was £800 per day, which grossly underestimates the current cost of care. Although at first glance this appears to be financially attractive, in the UK, the majority of level 3 beds operate at an occupancy of more than 90% and a bed released in a level 3 facility by transferring a patient to level 2 will be refilled promptly. Therefore, for this system to be credible more critical care resources need to be made available to fund and staff both level 2 and level 3 facilities.

There are no randomised controlled trials comparing the outcome of ICUs and weaning centres. However, results from European and US case series suggest that patients whose primary problem is ventilator dependence can be managed in less intensive step-down units facilitating a focus on ventilatory care and rehabilitation with one weaning bed required for every 20 ICU beds.[30] The most recent data are from a regional weaning centre in the UK.[31] This study followed up all the neuromuscular and chest wall disease, post-surgical and COPD patients admitted over a 4-year period. The important message from this study was that of the 153 patients referred with weaning delay and failure, around a third were decannulated and weaned completely from ventilatory support, a third required home ventilation and a third died before leaving hospital. Unfortunately, there were no data available for the total numbers referred. Survival was best in the neuromuscular patients, who were also the patients most likely to require home ventilation. Survival was worst in the post-surgical group, especially in patients with prolonged ICU stay prior to transfer.

Future Developments in Weaning

Automated weaning machines, using closed loop knowledge-based algorithms, aim to maintain a patient in the 'comfort zone' during the weaning process. This is achieved by the ventilator regularly monitoring respiratory rate, tidal volume and end-tidal carbon dioxide and gradually reducing the pressure support to a minimum at which stage the machine will automatically perform a SBT and deliver a message to inform the bedside nurse when the SBT has been successfully passed. Such ventilators are now available in mainstream clinical practice (Evita 4, Dräger, Lubeck, Germany), and data from preliminary studies show a benefit.[32] In the study by Lellouche et al., the computer-driven weaning arm, compared to the weaning guideline arm, had a reduction in weaning duration of 2 days and a decrease in total duration of mechanical ventilation of 4.5 days. However, the results of this study cannot be generalised to all patients as only 14% of eligible patients were randomised and thus more research is required. Nevertheless, since compliance with weaning protocols is frequently low,[3,24,33] computer-driven weaning could be a useful adjunct, especially in the early phases of weaning. In contrast to these advances in technology, we must also focus on the less technical aspects of caring for patients weaning from ventilation and, in particular, to those patients with weaning delay and weaning failure. There is now an increasing literature about the psychological factors and their influence on the weaning process. In a recent study by Wade et al.,[34] self-efficacy (coping ability) and positive emotion was a predictor of a patient's ability to wean, regardless of physiological parameters. It is therefore reasonable to hypothesise that enhancing the ability of the nurses and medical staff to communicate and provide psychological support to patients weaning from mechanical ventilation could impact on patients with weaning delay and weaning failure.

In conclusion, weaning is a complex challenging task. Critical care specialists must continually assess the readiness of patients to wean from mechanical ventilation and carefully evaluate the response to a reduction in ventilatory support. All units should adopt a flexible weaning practice with difficult-to-wean patients being identified early to optimise all physiological parameters. If problems are anticipated with weaning in patients with chronic lung, chest wall or neuromuscular disease, then an early referral to a weaning unit is advised.

References

1. Brochard L, Rauss A, Benito S, et al. Comparison of three methods of gradual withdrawal from ventilatory support during weaning from mechanical ventilation. *Am J Respir Crit Care Med.* 1994;150: 896–903.

2. Esteban A, Frutos F, Tobin MJ, et al. A comparison of four methods of weaning patients from mechanical ventilation. *N Engl J Med.* 1995;332:345–350.

3. Krishnan JA, Moore D, Robeson C, Rand CS, Fessler HE. A prospective, controlled trial of a protocol-based strategy to discontinue mechanical ventilation. *Am J Respir Crit Care Med.* 2004;169(6):673–678.

4. Make BJ. Indications for home ventilation. In: Robert D, Make BJ, Leger P, eds. *Home Mechanical Ventilation.* Paris: Arnette Blackwell; 1995:229–240.

5. Ely EW, Baker AM, Dunagan DP, et al. Effect on the duration of mechanical ventilation of identifying patients capable of breathing spontaneously. *N Engl J Med.* 1996;335(25):1864–1869.

6. Weaning and longterm ventilation: critical care programme. London: NHS Modernisation Agency; 2002.

7. Jubran A, Tobin MJ. Pathophysiological basis of acute respiratory distress in patients who fail a trial of weaning from mechanical ventilation. *Am J Respir Crit Care Med.* 1997;155:906–915.

8. Laghi F, Cattapan SE, Jubran A, et al. Is weaning failure caused by low-frequency fatigue of the diaphragm? *Am J Respir Crit Care Med.* 2003;167(2): 120–127.

9. Torres A, Aznar R, Gatell JM, et al. Incidence, risk, and prognosis factors of nosocomial pneumonia in mechanically ventilated patients. *Am Rev Respir Dis.* 1990;142(3):523–528.

10. Drakulovic MB, Torres A, Bauer TT, Nicolas JM, Nogué S, Ferrer M. Supine body position as a risk factor for nosocomial pneumonia in mechanically ventilated patients: a randomised trial. *Lancet.* 1999;354(9193):1851–1858.

11. Nava S, Rubini F, Zanotti E, et al. Survival and prediction of successful ventilator weaning in COPD patients requiring mechanical ventilation for more than 21 days. *Eur Respir J.* 1994;7(9):1645–1652.

12. Troche G, Moine P. Is the duration of mechanical ventilation predictable? *Chest.* 1997;112(3):745–751.

13. Esteban A, Alia I, Ibanez J, Benito S, Tobin, MJ. Modes of mechanical ventilation and weaning. A national survey of Spanish hospitals. The Spanish Lung Failure Collaborative Group. *Chest.* 1994;106(4): 1188–1193.

14. Esteban A, Alia I, Gordo F, et al. Extubation outcome after spontaneous breathing trials with T-tube or pressure support ventilation. The Spanish Lung Failure Collaborative Group. *Am J Respir Crit Care Med.* 1997;156(Suppl 2, pt 1): 459–465.

15. Epstein SK, Ciubotaru RL, Wong JB. Effect of failed extubation on the outcome of mechanical ventilation. *Chest.* 1997;112(1): 186–192.

16. Yang KL, Tobin MJ. A prospective study of indexes predicting the outcome of trials of weaning from mechanical ventilation. *N Engl J Med.* 1991;324(21): 1445–1450.

17. Sox HC, Jr. Probability theory in the use of diagnostic tests. An introduction to critical study of the literature. *Ann Intern Med.* 1986;104(1):60–66.

18. MacIntyre NR, Cook DJ, Ely EW Jr, et al. Evidence-based guidelines for weaning and discontinuing ventilatory support: a collective task force facilitated by the American College of Chest Physicians; the American Association for Respiratory Care; and the American College of Critical Care Medicine. Chest. 2001;120(Suppl 6):375S–395S.

19. Esteban A, Alia I, Tobin MJ, et al. Effect of spontaneous breathing trial duration on outcome of attempts to discontinue mechanical ventilation. Spanish Lung Failure Collaborative Group. *Am J Respir Crit Care Med.* 1999;159(2):512–518.

20. Kollef MH, Shapiro SD, Silver P, et al. A randomized, controlled trial of protocol-directed versus physician-directed weaning from mechanical ventilation. *Crit Care Med.* 1997;25(4):567–574.

21. Randolph AG, Wypij D, Venkataraman ST, et al. Effect of mechanical ventilator weaning protocols on respiratory outcomes in infants and children: a randomized controlled trial. *JAMA.* 2002;288(20): 2561–2568.

22. Namen AM, Ely EW, Tatter SB, et al. Predictors of successful extubation in neurosurgical patients. *Am J Respir Crit Care Med.* 2001;163(Suppl 3, pt 1):658–664.

23. Marelich GP, Murin S, Battistella F, Inciardi J, Vierra T, Roby M. Protocol weaning of mechanical ventilation in medical and surgical patients by respiratory care practitioners and nurses: effect on weaning time and incidence of ventilator-associated pneumonia. *Chest.* 2000;118(2):459–467.

24. Ely EW, Bennett PA, Bowton DL, Murphy SM, Florance AM, Haponik EF. Large scale implementation of a respiratory therapist-driven protocol for ventilator weaning. *Am J Respir Crit Care Med.* 1999;159(2):439–446.

25. Girault C, Daudenthun I, Chevron V, Tamion F, Leroy J, Bonmarchand G. Noninvasive ventilation as a systematic extubation and weaning technique in acute-on-chronic respiratory failure: a prospective, randomized controlled study. *Am J Respir Crit Care Med.* 1999;160(1):86–92.

26. Ferrer M, Esquinas A, Arancibia F, et al. Noninvasive ventilation during persistent weaning failure: a randomized controlled trial. *Am J Respir Crit Care Med.* 2003;168(1): 70–76.

27. Nava S, Ambrosino N, Clini E, et al. Noninvasive mechanical ventilation in the weaning of patients with respiratory failure due to chronic obstructive pulmonary disease. A randomized, controlled trial. *Ann Intern Med.* 1998;128(9):721–728.

28. Esteban A, Frutos-Vivar F, Ferguson ND, et al. Non-invasive positive-pressure ventilation for respiratory failure after extubation. *N Engl J Med.* 2004;350(24):2452–2460.

29. Robson V, Poynter J, Lawler PG, Baudouin SV. The need for a regional weaning centre, a one-year survey of intensive care weaning delay in the Northern Region of England. *Anaesthesia.* 2003;58(2): 161–165.

30. Simonds AK. Streamlining weaning: protocols and weaning units. *Thorax.* 2005;60(3):175–182.

31. Pilcher DV, Bailey MJ, Treacher DF, Hamid S, Williams AJ, Davidson AC. Outcomes, cost and long term survival of patients referred to a regional weaning centre. *Thorax.* 2005;60(3):187–192.

32. Lellouche F, Mancebo J, Jolliet P, et al. A multicenter randomized trial of computer-driven protocolized weaning from mechanical ventilation. *Am J Respir Crit Care Med.* 2006;174(8):894–900.

33. Iregui M, Ward S, Clinikscale D, Clayton D, Kollef MH. Use of a handheld computer by respiratory care practitioners to improve the efficiency of weaning patients from mechanical ventilation. *Crit Care Med.* 2002;30(9):2038–2043.

34. Wade D, Sherry T, Lei K, et al. An exploratory study of psychological factors in the process of weaning from mechanical ventilation. *Thorax.* 2007;62:A91.

Index

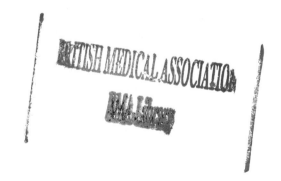